Stretching

The Best Exercises to Avoid Running Injuries

(Easy to Do Stretches Exercise Suitable for Both Men and Women)

Harold Irwin

Published By **Kate Sanders**

Harold Irwin

All Rights Reserved

Stretching: The Best Exercises to Avoid Running Injuries (Easy to Do Stretches Exercise Suitable for Both Men and Women)

ISBN   978-1-7770427-7-6

No part of this guidebook shall be reproduced in any form without permission in writing from the publisher except in the case of brief quotations embodied in critical articles or reviews.

Legal & Disclaimer

Upon using the information contained in this book, you agree to hold harmless the Author from and against any damages, costs, and expenses, including any legal fees potentially resulting from the application of any of the information provided by this guide. This disclaimer applies to any damages or injury caused by the use and application, whether directly or indirectly, of any advice or information presented, whether for breach of contract, tort, negligence, personal injury, criminal intent, or under any other cause of action.

You agree to accept all risks of using the information presented inside this book. You need to consult a professional medical practitioner in order to ensure you are both able and healthy enough to participate in this program.

Table Of Contents

Chapter 1: The Power Of Stretching

Stretching is a great manner for seniors to maintain flexibility and prevent damage. Regular stretching allows enhancing blood waft, reducing pressure, and increasing range of movement. Additionally, stretching can assist to ease joint ache and stiffness. Overall, incorporating stretching right right into a every day regular can drastically beautify senior's physical properly-being and extremely good of existence.

Stretching may want to have gigantic blessings for seniors, inclusive of advanced flexibility, sort of motion, and mobility. It also can lessen the danger of damage and help alleviate joint and muscle pain. Stretching often can also enhance posture and stability, making normal sports activities much less complicated and more secure. However, it's far important for seniors to be careful and not overdo it, as excessive stretching can result in muscle strain or other injuries. A mild stretching regular, done with right shape and below the steering of a healthcare expert, can be an effective manner for seniors to maintain and improve their bodily fitness.

Why Is It Important For Seniors To Stretch After A Long Day Of Work?

Many seniors might be surprised to discover how crucial it's miles for them to stretch out after operating all day. Although they'll now not recognize the proper technique, seniors who make the effort to stretch will see many advantages. Additionally, stretching can assist save you muscle aches and pains which may be commonplace with age and special bodily ailments that might make every day extra cushty for older adults. We'll cover a few motives why seniors want to find out time in their busy schedules to stretch day by day.

First of all, stretching engages muscle tissues in the end of your complete frame and permits counteract any stiffness or ache due to sitting at a table for hours on give up. Stretching moreover will boom your flexibility, in order to help you avoid damage

2

to your joints or muscle organizations. It's essential to encompass stretching into your day by day normal earlier than and while you start shifting spherical. You have to stretch as soon as you awaken within the morning in order that your body is limber whilst it enters into its lively duration inside the day. Additionally, you should include stretching on the prevent of each day to assist lighten up any tight muscle tissue after being seated for an extended time body.

How do seniors stretch properly?

Because seniors may be a good deal less bendy than more youthful humans, a mild shape of stretches is generally encouraged for them. When seniors perform stretches, they must be moderate, as they may locate it tough to move lower back to their actual characteristic. To accomplish this, the senior have to try to bend their knees as little as possible. For distinct varieties of stretching, which include a hamstring stretch or another time stretch, seniors must maintain their knees together and lean barely ahead even as preserving their backs right away.

How regularly is stretching endorsed for seniors?

Although it is not important to stretch every day, most older adults will gain from at the least   units of stretching sports activities constant with week. For this reason, it is exquisite in case you encompass stretches into your weekly recurring so that you can revel in the gain of advanced flexibility and lessening aches and pains within the method.

Which types of stretching are useful for older adults?

When seniors try and stretch, they should cognizance on lengthening and strengthening wearing sports that focus on the muscle companies of their our our bodies. Stretches have to be accomplished slowly and gently so that you can avoid any accidents. Some of the top notch stretches for seniors consist of sitting lower back, in that you slowly lean lower once more for your chair until a slight stretch is felt. Another first-rate stretch for seniors is to arise and gently reach for the sky, maintaining your palms out and arching your decrease again barely. Additionally, you can attempt stretching via putting one hand on a chair or wall and slowly attain behind you with the alternative hand to touch it.

Where want to seniors stretch?

Seniors who are interested in performing stretches should make sure they've got masses of room without any dangers close by to keep away from injuring themselves. It's additionally encouraged that seniors perform stretches even as fame in choice to sitting down because of the fact being seated can also cause muscle tightness. Seniors who carry out few or no stretches every week are at threat for some of physical illnesses, which consist of joint pain and muscle swelling. For this cause, stretching is crucial due to the fact it may assist decorate flexibility and save you the development of accidents.

How can a senior gain thru stretching?

Of direction, seniors won't enjoy the same advantages as more younger human beings due to the reality many seniors are lots a great deal less flexible than more youthful adults. However, as soon as you've got mastered primary stretches that focus on your decrease frame together with hamstring stretches or decrease lower back stretches, physical sports activities which encompass toe touch and crunches are great approaches to growth flexibility. Additionally, every yoga and tai chi provide incredible alternatives for seniors as a way to offer a boost in your muscle groups all through your frame even as assisting beautify flexibility within the approach.

IMPORTANCE OF WARM UP

Getting older is a great element. We are wiser and feature less to fear about than we did in our more youthful years, and it's easy to grow to be a piece complacent together with your fitness regular. But clearly because of the truth you are no longer a younger whippersnapper anymore would possibly not imply that you need to stop disturbing approximately your body! The reality is, as we age, our muscle mass broaden weaker and don't provide the same diploma of resource for the rest of our skeletal gadget. In order to keep your fitness as outstanding as feasible, you could want to offer your bodily health ordinary a piece TLC.

Warm up bodily activities are essential for seniors in advance than they interact in any physical interest as it enables to prepare their muscle companies and joints for the workout. A nicely heat-up routine can assist to boom blood flow, beautify sort of movement, reduce the danger of harm, and enhance famous performance. For seniors, a low-impact warm temperature-up, along with taking walks or mild stretching, is usually recommended to save you traces or sprains. It is critical to examine that warmth-americahave to be tailored to man or woman desires and competencies, so it's miles recommended to looking for advice from a healthcare professional in advance than starting any new exercising recurring.

In ultra-contemporary years, physical therapists and plenty of fitness experts have touted the benefits of stretching to assist older adults prevent harm. It is becoming more common understanding that in case you feel ache in any part of your frame, then you need to save you some element it's miles you're doing and take a warmth-up in advance than doing whatever new. So, why will we enjoy pain at the identical time as we do physical interest without warming up?

Before you begin your physical interest, you need to take a warmness up. This consists of moderate hobby on its very own, or doing the equal interest at a decrease intensity. In each case, it should increase the coronary heart charge and make you sweat barely. If the first-rate and comfy-up is simply too extreme for what you are approximately to do, you then truly definately are not getting the entire benefits of stretching before exercise. When you are ready to begin your hobby, you may use the equal normal that you commonly use. Using the same recurring is important because of the truth introducing a latest movement into your recurring can cause damage and can purpose confusion. So, if it's a electricity education software program in that you've been the use of the bench press for severa months, perhaps attempt doing it on an incline rather than flat, after which alternate with dumbbells.

Stretching is an critical a part of any workout and it have to be used in advance than your warm-up hobby. The National Athletic Trainers' Association recommends that people should do dynamic warm-u.S.To prepare their muscle groups for exercise. A dynamic warm-up is a warmness-up regular that focuses on a particular joint or muscle enterprise earlier than you begin your hobby.

The top notch time to stretch is earlier than you start an exercising or motion, no longer after. For instance, if you are going to begin a bench press exercising, do no longer do it right away. Instead, carry out a bit stretching first.

If you may stretch after your heat-up, then you may attention on your huge muscle organizations like your hamstrings and decrease decrease again. You must moreover stretch in between devices of exercising if you are lifting weights due to the reality the movement can positioned strain on the ones joints and muscle groups.

Stretching is crucial for seniors to hold right frame alignment and versatility. In addition to improving range of movement, it could reduce the risk of injury through developing flexibility, stability, manage and electricity. Stretching moreover assists with flow thru enhancing blood flow finally of our bodies; it is why it's important no longer sincerely to seniors but all of us. After all, in case you're no longer genuinely healthy you then in reality definately aren't going an amazing way to maintain a wholesome frame.

OUR BODIES AS WE AGE

Developing new approaches to take care of and decorate our physical appearance is a big, multi-billion greenback enterprise. With the growing older populace growing every one year, studies into splendor and durability is a rapidly evolving place. Technology has superior our clinical facts of the manner age influences the frame: telomeres that decide lifespan are clearly being understood in terms of nanometers; dermal fillers like Restylane, Juvederm, and Radiesse have progressed a person's pores and skin tone; even plastic surgical treatment has gotten much less invasive with the arrival of microblading. At this factor it is secure to mention that there aren't any limits on what we can reap on the equal time as we are developing older. All we need is time and staying power.

Aging Gracefully with General Wellness

One of the number one matters many humans do as they age is get their health checked. More and in addition, health experts have become advocates for preventative healthcare. With an getting older population, it is important that we deal with cutting-edge-day problems and modifications in our our bodies as we age to make sure more healthy lives. However, many doctors save you at recommending test-u.S.A.For coronary heart ailment and most cancers in choice to persevering with with substantial well-being visits throughout an elderly character's lifestyles.

There are a number of techniques to attend to ourselves as we age. Consuming give up end result, greens and healthful fat whilst warding off processed meals will assist gradual down the growing older technique, retaining your internal organs more wholesome longer. Exercise each day (preferably outside or with out using a gym), and get enough sleep, as strange sleep patterns contribute to a sophisticated chance of coronary coronary heart disease and plenty of one-of-a-kind illnesses.

Bleeding issues, mind fog, pressure, despair, reminiscence loss: all of these are symptoms that your hormones is probably out of whack. You can combat the ones commonplace signs with the aid of manner of creating small changes for your each day normal. Exercise is an excellent answer for almost every state of affairs, with advantages extending to cellular metabolism and DNA form. Next, get more sleep, plan to relax every day and address yourself to an occasional rub down. These small changes will make a big difference inside the frame's capability to heal itself.

IMPORTANCE OF EXERCISES

Exercise is crucial for the body and permits within the manufacturing of endorphins, which might be hormones to make you experience right. It enables in enhancing your temper. Exercise will can help you sleep higher at night time. It moreover strengthens your immune device with the beneficial aid of growing white blood cells which assist combat infection and decrease blood sugar stages, thereby preventing diabetes or a coronary heart assault. Also, it improves cardiovascular health via decreasing lousy ldl ldl cholesterol and growing right cholesterol levels similarly to strengthening bones with the discharge of calcium from muscle mass and stimulation of nerves that bring about strong muscular tissues. Finally, workout reduces strain with the useful resource of liberating hormones like serotonin that make one enjoy comfortable or a bargain less demanding .

Exercise additionally improves intellectual fitness. It will will let you study new subjects and beautify your awareness. It shapes your mind to be greater alert and improves reminiscence through means of making new mind cells grow in your older ones.

Chapter 2: Effects Of Workout On Body

The human frame consists of many one-of-a-kind varieties of cells, each performing particular talents. Exercise improves the functioning of maximum of those cells with the aid of way of growing their boom or interest stages. This is called secondary recuperation. The maximum generally affected cells are muscle (the principle detail of exercise muscle companies) and the bone marrow which produces purple blood cells . Other varieties of cells tormented by exercise are the coronary heart, lungs, immune tool and frightened device .

Other consequences of workout at the frame include:

There are two kinds of exercising – cardio and anaerobic. The cease end quit end result of aerobic workout is that the human frame burns fat . Anaerobic sporting sports reason lactic acid to be launched from muscle fibers, thereby growing the coronary coronary coronary heart charge and respiration fee.

However, the lactic acid isn't released with the beneficial aid of muscle cells but thru the muscle businesses themselves , because of this avoiding damage to at least one-of-a-kind tissues in the body . Both types of exercise produce strength, which is wanted for muscle companies to artwork, in spite of the fact that the effect on glucose tolerance is based totally upon upon which type of exercise changed into finished.

Focus on oxygen consumption and cardiovascular health can give up end result from each cardio and anaerobic sports sports. However, aerobic bodily video games produce the greatest growth in cardiovascular fitness. The purpose of aerobic sporting activities is to transport a massive amount of oxygen rapid to all cells during the frame thru growing the coronary coronary coronary heart fee and blood float .

Possible thing outcomes of exercise

The maximum common without delay aspect impact is muscle pain. This can also upward thrust up even as an individual engages in new exercising or will increase their intensity or period of physical interest . This is because of the truth at some stage in exercising, muscle fibers come to be torn, resulting in ache and contamination . Soreness also can be due to muscle imbalances. For instance, muscle mass near joints may get more potent than ones farther faraway from joints .

Other facet results include mood issues, tension, joint ache, surprising chest pains, indigestion (heartburn), menstrual cramps or despair . An growth in coronary heart fee inside the route of workout is ordinary and need to no longer be feared. However, if the coronary coronary heart looks like it's miles pumping faster than commonplace, check with a clinical health practitioner . High-intensity exercising can cause hypoxia (low oxygen degrees) in individuals who are ill or have kidney sickness .

UPPER BODY STRETCHES FOR SENIORS

There are primary types of stretches for the better frame, static and dynamic stretching. Static stretching is when a muscle movements in a unmarried function as you stretch it, on the identical time as a dynamic stretch is whilst a muscle moves and stretches simultaneously. The benefits of doing each styles of stretching are immoderate blood strain, reduced risk of damage during ordinary sports, and prolonged flexibility. Some seniors might not be snug doing whole-variety range arm motions as they aged due to arthritis or one-of-a-kind conditions that would make performing those moves uncomfortable or painful. These seniors and individuals who are extra flexible than others must now not be discouraged from doing dynamic stretches further to the higher body physical video games they do. All of those blessings however comply with for the ones seniors who're comfortable with the ones motions. Stretching is a common exercise for fitness fans, squaddies, athletes, and those in stylish. Everyone might also furthermore have their very own manner of stretching their muscle companies: moms stretch on the same time as wearing their child, squaddies stretch earlier than conflict, dancers perform stretches to boom flexibility and muscle electricity through motion patterns called "performances", and vehicle personnel take time to stretch a couple of instances an afternoon. These people are similar to you and me: we have got our very very own way of stretching to boom flexibility and save you damage. Stretching can be useful to older adults as it reduces threat of harm for the duration of normal sports activities, improves standard flexibility, can reduce signs and symptoms related to arthritis and different conditions, or even beautify performance. To beautify your flexibility the maximum commonplace way is thru static stretching. Stretching may additionally relieve pain in precise muscle tissues and joints, decrease stiffness or discomfort, boom sort of motion (ROM), lessen risk of harm, decorate ease of motion (ease), enhance overall performance, and prevent similarly damage from accidents. According to the International Sports Sciences

Association, static stretching (retaining stretches for 15-30 seconds at a time) is more powerful than dynamic stretching (preserve stretches for 10-15 seconds at a time). Due to the one-of-a-kind intensities of static and dynamic stretching, seniors with excessive ache need to awareness on static stretches. Some examples of static stretching are the chest stretch and triceps stretch. Many people have a false impression that doing an workout while you stretch is counterintuitive or volatile, but this will sincerely help boom your type of motion. When muscle companies are stretched prior to exercise they increase in period a good way to growth their capacity to perform an movement better.

SHOULDER ROLLS

To carry out shoulder rolls stretching for seniors, study the ones little by little instructions:

1.Sit or stand together along with your decrease once more immediately and chin parallel to the floor.

2.Gently inhale as you raise your shoulders up toward your ears, then exhale as you roll them lower once more and down.

three.Repeat this motion severa instances, aiming for a clean and controlled rolling movement.

4.If you revel in any pain or discomfort inside the route of this workout, save you right away.

That is the little by little way for shoulder rolls stretching for seniors.

CHEST EXPANDER

Here is a step-by using-step device for performing the chest expander stretch for seniors:

1.Begin with the resource of standing with ft shoulder-width apart and retaining a chest expander with each palms.

2.Raise your arms up at shoulder-top, retaining them parallel to the floor.

three.Exhale and slowly pull the chest expander aside, bringing your hands out to the rims on the equal time as retaining your palms at shoulder-pinnacle.

four.Hold the stretch for 10-15 seconds, feeling the stretch for your chest muscle tissues.

5.Slowly launch the stretch thru bringing your fingers decrease once more collectively inside the the front of your chest.

6.Repeat for two-three units of 10-15 repetitions, as desired.

Remember to commonly pay hobby on your frame and handiest stretch to a comfortable degree.

DOORWAY STRETCH

Here is a step-via manner of-step technique for the Doorway Stretch for seniors:

1.Stand in an open doorway, managing the frame.

2.Raise each palms so that your arms are resting at the door frame.

three.Step slightly beforehand with one foot, preserving your fingers on the frame for help.

four.Keep your lower back right now and lean in advance slightly until you experience a stretch on your chest and shoulders.

five.Hold the stretch for 15-30 seconds.

6.Repeat on the opposite foot.

TRICEPS STRETCH

To do a triceps stretch for seniors, have a look at these steps:

1.Stand up right away collectively together with your ft shoulder-width apart.

2.Bring your right arm up and bend it in the decrease again of your head so that your right hand is touching the middle of your lower returned.

three.Use your left hand to gently press down to your right elbow to increase the stretch.

4.Hold the stretch for 15-30 seconds.

5.Release the stretch and repeat on the possibility arm.

TRUNK TWIST

To perform a Trunk Twist stretch for seniors, follow these step-via-step instructions:

1.Sit on the floor collectively together with your legs prolonged immediately out in the front of you

2.Cross your left leg over your right leg, putting your left foot at the ground out of doors of your proper knee.

3.Place your proper hand on the ground within the lower back of your right buttock.

four.Bend your left elbow and vicinity your left forearm at the outside of your right knee.

five.Slowly twist your torso to the left as a ways as you could, the use of your left forearm to push against your right knee for delivered resistance.

6.Hold this stretch for 15-30 seconds.

7.Release the stretch and repeat on the other element, crossing your right leg over your left and twisting to the proper.

Remember to pay attention on your body and simplest stretch to the issue of moderate ache, now not pain.

SHOULDER BLADE SQUEEZE

To carry out the Shoulder Blade Squeeze Stretch for seniors, observe those steps:

1.Sit or upward thrust up immediately together in conjunction with your hands comfortable at your facets.

2.Gently squeeze your shoulder blades together, as even though you are trying to keep a small item amongst them.

3.Hold this characteristic for five-10 seconds.

4.Release the squeeze and lighten up your shoulders.

five.Repeat for 10-15 repetitions.

6.Take a damage and repeat the exercising for some unique set of 10-15 repetitions.

Remember to carry out this stretch slowly and lightly, and alter the depth as had to keep away from ache or pain.

NECK STRETCHES

Here are grade by grade neck stretches for seniors:

1.Sit or upward thrust up proper away together along with your shoulders snug.

2.Tilt your head to the right and maintain for 15-30 seconds.

3.Bring your head again to the middle and repeat on the left problem.

four.Slowly tilt your head ahead, bringing your chin closer to your chest, and maintain for 15-30 seconds.

five.Slowly raise your head once more as a whole lot as the middle.

6.Slowly tilt your head lower again, looking up in the path of the ceiling, and preserve for 15-30 seconds.

7.Bring your head lower once more to the center and repeat the complete series 2-three greater instances as desired.

WALL ANGELS

To perform the Wall Angels stretch for seniors, have a study these step-with the useful resource of manner of-step commands:

1.Stand going through a wall and place your heels about 6 inches some distance from it.

2.Lean lower back and press your lower returned towards the wall.

three.Make notable your hips, shoulders, and head are all touching the wall.

four.Bring your hands up, bending your elbows at a ninety-degree perspective, and phone your arms to the wall.

5.Slowly straighten your palms up, at the same time as keeping them in contact with the wall.

6.Once your hands are absolutely extended, slowly lower them go into reverse to the start position.

7.Repeat the movement for 10-15 reps, 2-three times a day.

Remember to take a while and bypass slowly and without problems through every step. Over time, you want to feel an improvement to your sort of movement and posture

Chapter 3: Shoulder Stretch

Here is a step-by means of-step method for a shoulder stretch that seniors can do:

1.Stand with your feet shoulder-width apart and your palms at your aspect.

2.Bring your right arm all through your chest, putting your left hand for your higher proper arm.

3.Hold for 20 to 30 seconds, feeling the stretch to your shoulder.

four.Repeat at the alternative aspect.

5.For an extra stretch, location your fingertips in your shoulders and rotate your elbows in circles.

6.Remember to not overstretch and pay attention for your frame.

UPPER BACK STRETCH

To perform an top once more stretch for seniors, look at those steps:

1.Begin in a seated role along side your toes flat on the floor.

2.Clasp your fingers together in front of your chest.

3.Round your top decrease returned and drop your chin to your chest.

four.Hold the stretch for 10-15 seconds, respiration deeply.

five.Release the stretch and gently roll your shoulders in a round movement.

6.Repeat the stretch 2-3 times or as preferred.

This stretch can help improve flexibility and reduce tension within the top once more muscle tissues.

NECK SIDE STRETCH

Here is a step-with the resource of-step machine for appearing the neck aspect stretch for seniors:

1.Sit upright in a snug chair together with your toes flat on the ground.

2.Begin with the useful resource of tilting your head to the right, gently bringing your right ear in the path of your right shoulder.

three.Hold the stretch for 15-30 seconds, feeling the stretch thru the left component of your neck.

four.Slowly bypass lower back your head to center.

five.Repeat on the left facet, bringing your left ear within the route of your left shoulder.

6.Hold the stretch for 15-30 seconds, feeling the stretch through the proper issue of your neck.

7.Return your head to center and repeat the whole collection 2-three times on each issue, as favored.

UPPER TRAPEZIUS STRETCH

Step with the useful useful resource of step device to do the better trapezius stretch for seniors:

1.Sit in a chair and keep your again straight away.

2.Looking right away earlier, tilt your head toward your left shoulder till you enjoy a stretch within the proper thing of your neck and higher shoulder.

3.Use your left hand to gently pull your head down inside the direction of your left shoulder.

four.Hold this feature for 10-15 seconds.

5.Release and pass again to the beginning feature, searching right away in advance.

6.Now tilt your head toward your proper shoulder until you feel a stretch within the left detail of your neck and higher shoulder.

7.Use your right hand to softly pull your head down within the route of your right shoulder.

8.Hold this function for 10-15 seconds.

9.Release and move returned to the beginning feature, searching instantly beforehand.

10. Repeat this stretch 2-three instances on each element.

Note: If you enjoy any ache or pain, save you the stretch straight away. Consult with a systematic expert when you have any issues.

CHEST STRETCH

Here is a step-thru-step manner for a chest stretch that seniors can do:

1.Stand tall collectively along with your spine proper away and feet shoulder-width apart.

2.Clasp your fingers inside the lower back of your returned.

three.Slowly decorate your hands as excessive as you may, keeping your elbows at once and your palms close to your frame.

4.Hold the stretch for 15-30 seconds.

five.Release your palms and loosen up your arms.

Remember to respire deeply and exhale as you stretch. You can repeat this stretch severa times sooner or later of the day as needed.

TRICEP STRETCH

Here is a grade by grade technique for Tricep stretch for seniors:

1.Start through reputation super and tall alongside facet your ft shoulder-width apart and your hands through your sides.

2.Lift your proper arm above your head collectively along with your palm going thru inwards toward your head.

3.Bend your elbow to hold your proper hand closer to your left shoulder blade.

four.Keep your elbow pointing at once as an awful lot as the ceiling and use your left hand to gently push your proper elbow deeper into the stretch.

five.Hold the stretch for 15-30 seconds and then release.

6.Repeat on the opposite component through the usage of lifting your left arm above your head.

SHOULDER BLADE SQUEEZE

Here is a step-via-step way for acting the shoulder blade squeeze:

1.Sit or stand along with your again immediately.

2.Reach your fingers out to the perimeters, together with your elbows bent at a 90-degree attitude.

3.Squeeze your shoulder blades collectively in the back of your once more.

4.Hold the squeeze for 5-10 seconds.

five.Release the squeeze and lighten up your shoulders.

6.Repeat the workout for 3 gadgets of 10-15 repetitions.

BICEP STRETCH

Here is a step-with the resource of using-step device for a bicep stretch that is secure for seniors:

1.Stand together in conjunction with your ft shoulder-width apart and hold your all over again immediately.

2.Raise your arms up in order that they may be straight away out in front of you, fingers dealing with down.

3.Slowly bend your elbows and produce your hands inside the route of your shoulders.

4.Hold the stretch for 10-15 seconds.

five.Slowly launch the stretch and produce your fingers backpedal on your sides.

6.Repeat the stretch 2-3 instances on each arm, resting for some seconds in amongst every stretch.

Remember to in no way push your self too difficult and to talk about collectively together with your medical scientific doctor before attempting any new workout normal.

QUAD STRETCH

To perform the quad stretch for seniors, comply with the ones steps:

1.Stand in the back of a chair or keep onto a wall for help.

2.Bend one leg over again on the knee, bringing your heel in the direction of your buttocks.

three.Use your hand to apprehend your ankle and gently pull it towards your buttocks.

4.Hold the stretch for 15 to 30 seconds, feeling the stretch in the front of your thigh.

five.Release the stretch and repeat at the opportunity leg.

WALL PUSH-UP

Step-with the beneficial aid of-step approach for wall push-u.S.A.For seniors:

1.Find a wall that is robust and flat.

2.Stand approximately ft far from the wall, collectively collectively together with your ft shoulder-width apart.

3.Place your hands flat in competition to the wall at shoulder height.

four.Slowly bend your elbows and lean your body in within the path of the wall, maintaining your once more instantly.

5.Pause while your nose nearly touches the wall.

6.Push your frame decrease again to the begin function.

7.Repeat steps four-6 for the popular variety of reps.

Note: If you have got any ache or ache on the equal time as doing wall push-ups, stop right away and speak over with a medical physician or healthcare professional.

WALL ANGELS

1.Stand with your again towards a wall, ft shoulder-width apart and approximately 6 inches some distance from the wall.

2.Lift your palms to shoulder top and bend your elbows to a 90-diploma mind-set, together along with your hands facing beforehand. This is your starting function.

3.Slowly slide your forearms up the wall, maintaining your elbows and wrists in touch with the wall always.

four.When you can't slide your fingers up any farther, hold the position for 10 to 30 seconds.

five.Slowly slide your forearms down the wall to go lower returned to the beginning position.

6.Repeat for the popular huge type of repetitions

WALL SLIDES

Here is a step-by means of manner of-step method for doing wall slides for seniors:

1.Begin via standing along facet your lower again toward a wall and your toes approximately shoulder-width apart.

2.Slowly slide your hands up the wall, preserving your elbows without delay and your shoulders down.

3.When you attain the factor in which you sense a stretch on your shoulders, pause for a few seconds.

4.Slowly decrease your fingers go into reverse to the beginning role.

five.Repeat this movement for 10-12 repetitions.

Remember to move slowly and intentionally, and forestall proper now if you experience any pain or pain.

WALL PLANK

1.Begin with the resource of choosing a sturdy wall this is free of limitations, which encompass fixtures or different decorative gadgets.

2.Hold the plank in opposition to the wall, with your fingers shoulder-width aside and your legs hip-width apart. Your body need to form a directly line out of your head to your heels.

three.Engage your middle muscle organizations by way of using pulling your belly button in the direction of your spine. Make first rate to keep your hips ordinary along side your shoulders.

4.Hold the plank for 10-30 seconds, or so long as you could without compromising proper shape. Remember to respire step by step at some point of the exercising.

five.Repeat the workout for 3-4 gadgets, resting for 30-60 seconds amongst each set.

6.As you improvement, you could increase the length of each plank keep or contain versions such as aspect planks or mountain climbers. Always be aware of your frame and are in search of advice from a fitness professional if you experience any pain or ache.

LAT STRETCH

Here is a step-through manner of-step technique for seniors to do a lat stretch:

1.Stand collectively together together with your ft hip-distance apart and parallel to every distinct.

2.Reach your right arm up toward the ceiling. three.Bend your proper elbow and vicinity your right hand for your again, just above your waist.

four.Take your left hand and place it at the outside of your proper elbow.

5.Gently pull your right elbow in the direction of your left issue, until you experience a stretch in your proper lat muscular tissues.

6.Hold the stretch for 15-30 seconds.

Chapter 4: Lower Body Stretches For Seniors

A lot of humans over the age of sixty five begin to experience joint ache. For the ones seniors, it's miles crucial to be cognizant of this reality and do what they will to keep away from making the pain worse. This may be as clean as some stretches or as difficult as buy orthotics for his or her footwear, but a hint bit is going an prolonged manner in preventing chronic ache.

When first considering decrease body stretches for seniors, it's far vital to apprehend the way that this population actions. Many seniors have problems with stability and as such, have a incredible deal of problem with taking walks. So even as we are saying that most people over sixty 5 years old need to stretch their decrease our bodies, we advocate their hamstrings and calves. These are muscle groups which might be used at some stage in on foot and if they will be in ache, seniors may not skip in any respect.

Balance is an hassle for plenty seniors then you without a doubt ought to moreover think about how this influences the manner that you glide spherical your private home. If you have were given a senior residing with you, you apprehend the worrying situations that they will be dealing with sooner or later of the day. You ought to likely need to put in snatch rails and hand holds in regions of your private home wherein stability is a subject. Including some decrease body stretches for seniors wherein they'll be able to grab onto some element if wanted will help them to transport spherical more and not using a hassle and correctly

Lower frame stretches for seniors are greater generally practiced than you accept as true with you studied. The maximum apparent example is yoga. While they will no longer be capable of perform all the poses, any stretching that they're capable of do indoors their limits is going to help them maintain their variety of movement and save you loads of ache later on when they do want to do some component active.

SEATED TOE TOUCHES

Begin seated toe touches for senior via following the grade by grade device below:

1.Sit on a sturdy chair along with your lower back proper away, feet flat on the ground and hip-width aside.

2.Place your fingers on your thighs or knees and take a deep breath in.

three.As you exhale, slowly bend ahead out of your hips, bringing your chest in the direction of your knees.

four.Reach to your toes together with your fingers. If you can't obtain your feet, just stretch inside the direction of them as far as you can without straining.

five.Hold the stretch for 10-15 seconds after which slowly sit down down decrease again up.

6.Repeat the stretch 5-10 instances, taking deep breaths in among every set.

STANDING QUAD STRETCH

Here are step by step commands for the Standing Quad Stretch for seniors:

1.Stand tall collectively along with your toes hip-distance apart.

2.Using your proper hand, deliver your right foot off the ground and produce it within the direction of your buttocks.

three.Reach once more along side your left hand and hold close your right ankle or foot.

four.Gently pull your foot towards your buttocks until you enjoy a stretch to your quadricep muscle.

five.Hold the stretch for 10-30 seconds.

6.Release the stretch and repeat together at the side of your left leg.

SEATED LEG LIFTS

Step-with the resource of the usage of-step method for Seated Leg Lifts for seniors:

1.Sit in a chair collectively together with your decrease back without delay and toes flat on the ground.

2.Lift your right leg off the ground at the equal time as retaining it immediately.

3.Hold for some seconds after which decrease your leg back off.

4.Repeat collectively collectively together with your left leg.

five.Aim for 10-15 leg lifts on each leg, frequently growing the big variety as your energy improves.

6.Remember to breathe regularly sooner or later of the exercising.

SEATED LATERAL LEG STRETCH

Here is the little by little way for Seated Lateral Leg Stretch for seniors:

1.Sit on a chair on the aspect of your back instantly and feet flat on the floor.

2.Lift your left leg and region your foot on the outdoor of your right knee.

three.Place your left hand in your left knee and your proper hand for your ankle.

four.Inhale, sit up tall and prolong your spine.

5.Exhale, gently twist your torso to the left on the same time as using your left hand to press towards your left knee to deepen the stretch.

6.Hold for about 30 seconds.

7.Inhale, come decrease lower back to the center.

8.Exhale, slowly launch the stretch.

nine.Repeat at the opportunity element.

Remember to transport slow and in no manner stress the stretch, if you revel in any pain or pain, launch the stretch proper now.

STANDING GLUTE STRETCH

To perform a status glute stretch for seniors, follow the ones step-with the resource of-step instructions:

1.Begin via using recognition together with your toes hip-distance apart and your palms resting in your hips.

2.Take a breakthrough collectively with your left foot and shift your weight onto your left foot.

3.Bend your left knee slightly and lift your right foot off the floor.

4.Bring your right ankle up and vicinity it on your left knee, certainly above the knee joint.

five.Slowly lower your hips down and all over again as in case you have been sitting in a chair. You have to feel a stretch in your proper glute.

6.Hold the stretch for 15-30 seconds.

7.Return to a standing position and repeat at the opportunity factor.

Make powerful to maintain your lower back proper away and your center engaged throughout the stretch. If desired, you may use a chair or wall for balance.

STANDING HAMSTRING STRETCH

Step-via-step approach for Standing Hamstring Stretch for senior:

1.Stand in an upright feature together with your toes shoulder-width aside.

2.Extend one leg earlier and vicinity your heel at the ground.

three.With your fingers on your hips, gently lean in advance on the hips.

four.Hold the stretch for 10-30 seconds.

five.Release and repeat with the opposite leg.

6.Continue to trade stretching each leg for a total of 5-10 repetitions.

STANDING CALF STRETCH

Here are the step by step commands for the Standing Calf Stretch for seniors:

1.Place your fingers on a wall or particular robust floor.

2.Step lower lower back with one leg, preserving the knee proper now.

3.Press the heel of your lower returned foot into the ground.

four.Hold for 10-30 seconds.

five.Repeat with the opportunity leg.

SEATED BUTTERFLY STRETCH

Here is the step-with the useful resource of the usage of-step way for Seated Butterfly Stretch for seniors:

1.Sit at the floor together along side your lower back right away and your legs out in the the front of you.

2.Bend your knees and produce the soles of your feet together.

3.Use your palms to softly pull your toes within the path of your groin vicinity.

four.Hold the stretch for 10-30 seconds while respiration deeply.

5.Release the stretch and repeat as desired.

Remember to in no way pressure your body right into a stretch and to continually pay attention to your body's limits.

STAFF POSE

To carry out the personnel pose stretch for seniors step by step, observe those instructions:

1.Sit on a mat collectively together with your legs prolonged in the front of you.

2.Engage your thigh muscular tissues and press your legs into the mat.

3.Flex your toes and press via your heels.

four.Inhale and raise your fingers overhead.

five.Exhale and hinge ahead from the hips, accomplishing your arms in the direction of your toes.

6.Keep your backbone lengthy and your shoulders comfortable.

7.Hold the pose for severa breaths.

8.To release, inhale and sit up tall.

STANDING HIP FLEXOR STRETCH

Here is a step-by way of-step machine for the Standing Hip Flexor Stretch for seniors:

1.Begin fame with a chair or wall close by for assist.

2.Place your left foot on the ground in front of you, bending the knee.

3.Keep your right foot decrease again, in conjunction with your heel at the floor and feet pointing in advance.

four.Tighten your abs and glutes to keep proper posture.

5.Slowly lean ahead towards your left knee till you revel in a stretch on your right hip flexor.

6.Hold the stretch for 15-30 seconds.

7.Slowly launch the stretch and switch legs, repeating on the alternative element.

8.Remember to respire deeply and relax your shoulders at a few stage inside the stretch.

Note: If you sense any pain or pain during the stretch, forestall proper away and are looking for recommendation from a scientific expert.

BUTTERFLY STRETCH

Here is a step-via-step way for the Butterfly stretch for seniors:

1.Sit at the floor along side your legs extended inside the front of you.

2.Bend your knees and produce your feet together, so the soles of your feet touch.

3.Using your fingers, pull your heels toward your body, as close to as comfortable.

4.Hold onto your ankles or toes together along with your arms.

five.Gently press your elbows down onto your legs, feeling the stretch on your hips.

6.Hold the stretch for 15-30 seconds.

7.Release the stretch and go back on your starting function.

eight.Repeat the stretch 2-three greater instances, as snug.

Remember to take deep breaths in some unspecified time in the future of the stretch to help lighten up and amplify the muscle mass.

UPWARD DOG AND DOWNWARD DOG

Here is a step-with the resource of-step system to perform those stretches:

1.Begin for your hands and knees along side your fingers located virtually slightly in the the front of your shoulders.

2.Exhale and push up through your palms and raise your pelvis and thighs off the ground.

3.Keep your arms right away and your palms shoulder-width aside. Make excellent that your shoulders live a long way from your ears.

4.Lift your chest up in the route of the ceiling and gaze toward the sky.

five.Hold this position for some seconds, then exhale and launch go into reverse on your hands and knees.

6.To perform the Downward Dog stretch, maintain your arms and ft inside the identical positions as the Upward Dog role.

7.Exhale and lift your pelvis and hips up in the direction of the ceiling.

eight.Straighten your legs and arms as a superb deal as viable even as retaining your head and neck cushty.

nine.Press your heels closer to the floor and preserve this function for a few seconds.

10. Release backtrack to your fingers and knees to complete the stretch.

Remember to respire effortlessly and take it sluggish with each movement. It's critical to pay attention to your body and keep away from any motion that motives discomfort.

SEATED HIP STRETCH

Step with the useful resource of step approach for seated hip stretch for seniors:

1.Sit together collectively together with your lower back right now in a comfortable chair.

2.Place your ft flat on the floor, about hip-width apart.

three.Place your left ankle for your right knee, and lightly press down for your left knee at the facet of your left hand.

4.Hold this stretch for about 30 seconds, or as long as feels comfortable for you.

5.Switch sides and repeat collectively together together with your right ankle resting to your left knee.

6.Repeat this stretch on each factor 2-3 instances at a few degree in the day.

SEATED FORWARD BEND

To perform a seated in advance bend for seniors, look at those step by step commands:

1.Sit on a sturdy chair together along with your toes flat at the floor and your knees hip-width aside.

2.Place your hands on your thighs and take a deep breath in.

3.As you exhale, slowly start to lean beforehand from your hips, retaining your again straight away.

Chapter 5: Hip Opener

Here are the steps to do the hip opener stretch for seniors:

1.Begin by means of sitting on a yoga mat collectively in conjunction with your legs stretched out inside the the the front of you.

2.Slowly bend your right knee and convey it toward your chest.

three.Cross your proper ankle over your left knee.

4.Use your palms to softly press your right knee down inside the course of the ground.

5.Hold the stretch for 15-30 seconds, respiration deeply.

6.Release the stretch and repeat on the alternative aspect.

7.Repeat the stretch multiple times as preferred, little by little growing the length of the maintain if comfortable.

STANDING LUMBAR STRETCH

Step by way of way of step method for fame lumbar stretch for seniors:

1.Stand along side your ft shoulder-width apart, retaining your knees slightly bent.

2.Clasp each hands collectively within the lower back of your once more, near your hips.

three.Raise your fingers a long way from your all over again, accomplishing upward as far as cushty.

4.Gently bend ahead at your waist, keeping your knees bent and your palms above your hips.

five.Hold this stretch for 15-30 seconds, feeling a stretch for your decrease decrease decrease back.

6.Slowly come lower once more as a lot as a standing characteristic.

7.Repeat steps 2-6 for 2-three more repetitions.

SEATED KNEE TO CHEST STRETCH

1.Sit on a chair together along with your back immediately.

2.Place every toes flat at the floor and about hip distance apart.

three.Lift your right foot off the floor and loop a strap or towel across the most effective of your foot.

four.Slowly pull your proper knee in the path of your chest the use of the towel or strap until you enjoy a gentle stretch for your lower once more and hip.

5.Hold the stretch for 20-30 seconds.

6.Release your proper leg decrease lower back to the beginning position and repeat collectively with your left leg.

7.Do 2-3 units of 10-15 reps on each leg, each day or as encouraged with the useful resource of using your healthcare company.

KNEELING HIP FLEXOR STRETCH

Here is a step by step machine for the kneeling hip flexor stretch for seniors:

1.Begin in a kneeling characteristic on a mat or smooth surface.

2.Step your proper foot in advance, maintaining your knee bent at a ninety-degree mind-set.

3.Place your arms for your hips or relaxation them on your right thigh for help.

four.Ensure that your left knee is without difficulty resting at the ground

five.Gently shift your weight beforehand, pushing your pelvis forward until you sense a stretch for your left hip flexor.

6.Hold the stretch for 20-30 seconds.

7.Release the stretch and transfer facets, repeating the way together along with your left foot beforehand.

Remember to breathe deeply and pay interest in your body in some unspecified time within the destiny of the stretch. If you revel in any ache or discomfort, ease lower again at the stretch or forestall altogether.

MORNING STRETCH

Many senior citizens begin the day with a everyday morning stretch, which lets in to boom mobility and decrease ache in joints. Stretching bloodless muscle groups earlier than interest can assist save you harm at some degree inside the day. It can also additionally relieve tension for your frame that builds up over time.

It's clean to make morning stretches a part of your developing older habitual, however do no longer depend on them to healing slight or mild troubles consisting of decrease decrease decrease returned ache or arthritis stiffness. For these situations, speak to your medical doctor about what else you could do for consolation, which consist of taking up-the-counter ibuprofen or using an ice percent on sore joints. You furthermore may furthermore need to see a bodily therapist who focuses on treating older adults or a health practitioner who makes a speciality of treating arthritis-associated conditions.

What are the blessings of morning stretches for seniors?

Stretching can assist prevent muscle stiffness, decorate your sort of motion, and improve your strength level. The American Academy of Orthopaedic Surgeons recommends that you stretch:

NECK STRETCH

Here is the grade by grade technique to carry out neck stretches for seniors:

1. Sit in a snug feature together along with your again proper away.

2. Tilt your head slowly to the right, in search of to touch your ear to the shoulder on the same time as keeping your shoulders snug. Hold this function for 10-15 seconds.

3. Return your head to the middle and repeat the stretch at the left factor.

4. Now, drop your chin down in the direction of your chest and hold for 10-15 seconds.

five. Lift your chin upwards and look in the route of the ceiling, at the equal time as maintaining your shoulders down. Hold for 10-15 seconds.

6. Finally, flip your head slowly to the left as a protracted way as you can with out a trouble pass without straining. Hold for 10-15 seconds. Repeat on the right facet.

Remember to respire deeply for the duration of the stretches and save you at once in case you enjoy any ache.

SHOULDER SHRUG

Shoulder shrug for senior step by step method:

1. Stand or sit up straight together at the side of your fingers at your sides.

2. Slowly enhance your shoulders up towards your ears as immoderate as you can skip.

3. Hold for a second or .

four. Slowly lower your shoulders back off to their beginning characteristic.

5. Repeat for preferred quantity of reps.

ARM STRETCH

Arm Stretch for Seniors Step via Step Process:

1. Sit effortlessly in a chair alongside aspect your ft flat on the floor.

2. Interlock your arms and bring your hands up above your head, together with your arms dealing with upward.

three. Stretch your palms up as excessive as you can and keep the placement for ten seconds.

four. Slowly decrease your arms go into reverse on your aspects.

5. Repeat the stretch 5 to 10 times.

UPPER BODY TWIST

Step by the usage of the usage of step approach for higher body twist for seniors:

1. Sit upright in a chair along side your toes flat on the ground.

2. Keep your decrease back right away and your shoulders cushty.

3. Place your fingers to your hips and inhale deeply.

four. As you exhale, twist your better body to the right.

five. Hold this characteristic for some seconds, then inhale and go back to center.

6. Exhale and twist your higher body to the left.

7. Hold this role for a few seconds, then inhale and move again to middle.

8. Repeat this twisting movement for a few minutes, regularly developing the range of

movement if cushty.

nine. Remember to respire deeply at a few stage inside the exercising.

WRIST AND FINGER FLEX

1. Start through extending your arm right away out within the the front of your body.

2. Slowly bend your wrist upward until you experience a stretch to your forearm.

3. Hold the stretch for a few seconds.

four. Without letting pass of the stretch to your wrist, curl your hands inward as though developing a fist.

five. Hold the stretch for your wrist and fingers for some seconds.

6. Release the stretch to your palms and wrist, bringing your hands once more to their specific function.

7. Repeat the whole method 5-10 times on every hand.

HIP STRETCH

Here's a little by little manner for doing a hip stretch:

1. Begin through status together with your feet shoulder-width aside, making sure your spine is straight away.

2. Take a big leap forward at the side of your proper foot and bend your right knee at a ninety-degree perspective.

three. Keeping your left leg at once, shift your weight onto your right foot and lean forward barely.

4. Place every hands to your proper knee, maintaining your once more immediately and your chest upright.

5. Hold this role for 15-30 seconds, feeling the stretch on your left hip flexor.

6. Repeat steps 2-5 on the other facet, taking a large breakthrough together with your left foot.

Remember to breathe deeply sooner or later of the stretch and in no way push yourself past your limits. Consult with a systematic professional when you have any issues about acting stretches accurately.

HAMSTRING STRETCH

Here is a step-by means of manner of-step way for performing a hamstring stretch:

1. Sit at the floor with each legs at once out in the the the front of you.

2. Bend your right knee and location your proper foot flat on the ground next on your left thigh.

Chapter 6: Ankle Circles

To perform ankle circles as a stretching exercise:

1.Sit on a comfortable ground together together with your legs stretched out inside the the front of you.

2.Lift your proper foot off the floor and rotate your ankle clockwise in a round movement.

3.Perform 10 circles after which repeat in a counterclockwise course.

4.Repeat together collectively with your left foot.

5.Gradually boom your kind of motion because the exercise turns into a good deal less tough.

Note: Stop the workout in case you experience any ache or ache in your ankles. Consult with a systematic doctor when you have a data of ankle injuries.

LAYING DOWN STRETCHES

KNEE-TO-CHEST STRETCH

Here is the step-by way of way of the use of-step device for seniors to perform the knee-to-chest stretch:

1.Lie for your once more on a mat or comfortable floor collectively together with your legs extended.

2.Bend your proper knee and pull it inside the direction of your chest the use of every fingers clasped under your knee.

three.Hold your proper knee close to your chest for 10-30 seconds.

4.Return your right leg to the start feature.

5.Repeat steps 2-4 together along with your left leg.

6.Repeat the whole collection 2-four times for every leg.

GLUTE STRETCH

Here is a step-via the use of-step method for a glute stretch for seniors:

1.Sit on a sturdy chair at the side of your feet shoulder-width apart and flat on the ground.

2.Cross your proper ankle over your left knee.

three.Lean beforehand slightly at the same time as maintaining your lower once more directly.

four.You want to enjoy a stretch to your proper glute muscle.

five.Hold for 30 seconds.

6.Repeat on the alternative side through crossing your left ankle over your proper knee.

INNER THIGH STRETCH

Here's the step-with the useful resource of-step manner for inner thigh stretch for seniors:

1.Sit at the ground along with your legs stretched out inside the front of you.

2.Bend your left leg and convey your left foot inside the path of your right internal thigh.

three.Keep your right leg right away and slowly bend ahead from your hips in the route of your right leg.

4.Hold for 10-30 seconds.

five.Repeat at the opportunity facet.

PIRIFORMIS STRETCH

Here is a grade by grade way for Piriformis stretch for seniors:

1.Lie down to your again together together with your knees bent.

2.Cross your proper ankle over your left knee.

3.Use your fingers to softly pull your left knee in the direction of your chest.

four.Hold the stretch for 15-30 seconds.

five.Repeat at the opportunity element by manner of way of crossing your left ankle over your right knee.

6.Perform the stretch 2-3 instances on every side.

IT BAND STRETCH

Here's a grade by grade system for a IT band stretch for seniors:

1. Stand along side your left facet going thru a wall.

2. Cross your right leg inside the the the front of your left leg.

3. Lean your proper hip in opposition to the wall.

four. Slowly make bigger your left arm over your head, retaining your left hip pressed toward the wall.

5. Hold the stretch for 15-30 seconds.

6. Repeat on the alternative issue.

Note: This stretch want to be completed gently and regularly. If you enjoy any ache or ache, save you right now.

UPPER BACK STRETCH

Here are the grade by grade instructions for an better again stretch for seniors:

1.Sit in a chair together together together with your toes firmly planted on the floor and your again right away.

2.Clasp your arms collectively in the front of your chest along facet your arms managing inward.

three.Slowly make bigger your fingers ahead while protective onto your palms until you experience a stretch on your upper again.

four.Hold the stretch for 10-15 seconds and then launch.

five.Repeat the stretch 2-three times.

LOWER BACK STRETCH

Here is a grade by grade gadget for a decrease again stretch this is secure for seniors:

1.Lie down flat in your returned on a cushty floor, which incorporates a yoga mat or a carpeted ground.

2.Bend your knees and vicinity your toes flat on the floor.

three.Slowly deliver your knees up toward your chest, the use of your fingers to aid your legs and produce them towards your frame. Keep your head and shoulders flat in the direction of the floor.

4.Take a deep breath and hold this position for 10-15 seconds, feeling the stretch on your lower lower returned and hips.

five.Exhale and launch the stretch, extending your legs once more to the beginning function.

6.Repeat the stretch 2-3 times, taking breaks in amongst to rest and breathe. Remember to transport slowly and not push your frame past its limits.

COBRA POSE

To perform the Cobra pose stretch for seniors, follow the ones steps:

1.Lie down on your stomach collectively along with your fingers flat on the ground by using manner of your shoulders.

2.Inhale and gently raise your chest and shoulders off the ground the usage of your decrease again muscle corporations.

3.Keep your elbows near your body and your forearms flat on the floor.

4.Hold this pose for 15-30 seconds at the same time as breathing deeply.

five.To release, exhale and lightly decrease your chest and shoulders backtrack to the floor.

POSTURE STRETCHES

Chapter 7: Chest Opener

To carry out the chest opener stretch for seniors, have a examine those step-through-step commands:

1.Sit on the threshold of a chair with right posture and your toes flat at the ground.

2.Clasp your palms within the once more of your decrease once more, interlocking your arms.

three.Inhale deeply and, as you exhale, gently convey your hands up and far out of your frame.

four.Keep your chest and chin lifted, and look proper away ahead.

five.Hold the stretch for 15-30 seconds.

6.Slowly launch and go back your palms for your sides.

7.Repeat the stretch 2-three times, taking deep breaths in between.

FORWARD FOLD

The in advance fold stretch is a extraordinary manner for seniors to stretch their hamstrings. Here is a step-with the useful resource of manner of-step device:

1.Start via manner of fame up directly alongside facet your toes hip-width apart.

2.Take a deep breath in and lift your palms up overhead.

3.As you breathe out, gently bend ahead from the hips and reach down within the direction of the floor. Keep your knees barely bent and your again at once.

4.Place your palms to your shins, ankles, or the floor, depending in your flexibility.

5.Take some deep breaths in this feature, feeling the stretch in your hamstrings.

6.Slowly roll as a lot as a standing function, one vertebra at a time, and repeat as preferred.

TRUNK ROTATION

Here is a step-by using manner of using-step method for trunk rotation stretches for seniors:

1.Sit on a chair together together with your ft flat at the floor and your decrease again immediately.

2.Place your arms in your shoulders.

3.Slowly twist your better frame to the right, the usage of your middle muscle mass to rotate your backbone.

four.Hold the position for 10-15 seconds.

five.Return to the start function.

6.Repeat the stretch via rotating your body to the left.

7.Complete 10-15 repetitions on each aspect, or as directed with the aid of using your healthcare agency.

Remember to respire outside and inside slowly and deeply at some stage in the workout. If you revel in any pain or ache, prevent the stretch right now and attempting to find recommendation out of your scientific health practitioner.

MORE STRETCHES FOR SENIORS

LOCUST POSE

Here's a step-through-step method for doing the Locust Pose Stretch for seniors:

1.Lie flat in your belly on a snug and strong ground, preferably a yoga mat.

2.Bring your arms through your factors, together with your hands handling down and your brow resting at the mat.

3.With your legs collectively, have interaction your middle and lift your legs off the ground, preserving them without delay.

4.As you increase your legs, additionally increase your chest off the ground, stretching your higher frame.

five.Hold this characteristic for 10-30 seconds, breathing deeply and lightly.

6.Slowly release the stretch via lowering your legs and chest backtrack to the floor.

7.Repeat the stretch 2-three times, steadily growing the quantity of time you maintain the stretch as your body gets greater snug with it.

Remember to be aware about your frame, and if at any component you feel discomfort or pain, slowly release the stretch and take a damage earlier than attempting again.

RHOMBOID STRETCH

Here's a step-with the useful resource of way of-step way for seniors to do the rhomboid stretch:

1.Sit on a chair and location your arms in the decrease lower back of your head.

2.Squeeze your shoulder blades together and keep for 10 seconds.

three.Release and repeat for 10 repetitions.

four.Alternatively, you could stand and clasp your palms at the back of your decrease again, then boom your arms up and far from your body to stretch your rhomboids.

Remember to respire deeply and handiest stretch to a degree of mild soreness, no longer pain.

WRIST AND FOREARM STRETCH

Step thru step system for wrist and forearm stretch for seniors:

1.Sit in a cushty chair together collectively with your back immediately and feet flat at the ground.

2.Place your fingers right now out inside the the front of you collectively along with your palms dealing with down.

three.Raise your palms closer to the ceiling, maintaining your hands immediately, until you experience a stretch on your wrists and forearms.

four.Hold the stretch for 10-15 seconds.

five.Lower your palms backtrack to the begin function.

6.Repeat steps three-5 for an entire of three-4 times.

BACK STRETCH

To carry out a decrease lower lower back stretch for seniors, observe those steps:

1.Start via reputation together collectively together with your feet shoulder-width apart and maintaining your knees barely bent.

2.Place your arms for your decrease decrease again, along with your arms pointing downwards.

3.Slowly lean returned, arching your lower lower back and allowing your hands to guide your weight.

four.Hold this selection for 10-30 seconds.

5.Slowly skip again to the start position and repeat as vital.

Remember to move slowly and avoid any unexpected actions that would motive harm. It's moreover vital to are seeking out recommendation from a healthcare expert in advance than beginning any new workout regular.

LUNGE STRETCH

Here is a step-with the beneficial useful resource of-step device for performing the lunge stretch for seniors:

1.Stand up without delay together together together with your feet shoulder-width aside.

2.Take a soar ahead with one foot, making sure to keep your knee right away above your ankle.

three.Lower your again knee down inside the direction of the floor, whilst maintaining your the the front knee at a 90-degree mind-set.

four.Hold this characteristic for 10 to 30 seconds.

five.Slowly stand again up and repeat on the other aspect.

Remember to breathe deeply in the route of the stretch and to stop right away in case you experience pain.

ANKLE STRETCH

Here's a step-with the useful resource of the usage of-step method for seniors on a manner to do an ankle stretch:

1.Sit on a chair or bench together with your ft flat at the ground.

2.Place your right ankle for your left knee.

3.Gently press down on your proper knee to stretch the ankle.

4.Hold the stretch for 15-30 seconds.

five.Release the stretch and repeat with the possibility ankle.

6.Complete 2-three units on each ankle.

Remember to breathe deeply sooner or later of the stretch and prevent if you enjoy any ache.

SEATED SPINAL TWIST

Here is a grade by grade technique for the seated spinal twist for seniors:

1.Sit on a chair at the side of your feet flat on the floor.

2.Place your left hand on your right knee and your proper hand in the back of the chair.

3.Inhale and extend your backbone, accomplishing the crown of your head closer to the ceiling.

4.Exhale and lightly twist to the right, using your palms for manual.

five.Hold the pose for some breaths, preserving your spine tall and your shoulders snug.

6.On an inhale, release the twist and are available lower back to middle.

7.Repeat on the other component, setting your proper hand on your left knee and your left hand on the again of the chair.

Remember to pay hobby in your body and fine skip as a long way as feels snug for you.

Chapter 8: Seated Leg Extension

Here is a step-by using using-step technique for doing seated leg extensions for seniors:

1.Sit on a strong chair together along with your over again right away and your ft flat on the floor.

2.Slowly increase one leg right away out in front of you, extending it as a protracted manner as snug.

three.Hold the position in quick, then slowly decrease your leg go into reverse to the start function.

four.Repeat the manner on the facet of your specific leg.

five.Do 10-15 repetitions for each leg, and then rest for a minute.

6.Repeat the set 2-three times for a whole workout.

SEATED KNEE TUCK

Here is a step-by using-step system for seated leg extensions appropriate for seniors:

1.Sit on a robust chair collectively with your returned at once and your toes flat at the ground.

2.Extend one leg out inside the front of you, retaining it right now however no longer locking your knee.

three.Hold the prolonged function for 2-3 seconds.

four.Slowly decrease your leg back down to the start function.

5.Repeat at the side of your outstanding leg.

6.Aim for 10-15 repetitions on each leg, and steadily growth as you feel cushty.

Remember to respire frequently at some point of the workout, and prevent in case you enjoy any ache or pain. It is constantly endorsed to visit a healthcare expert in advance than starting any new exercise everyday.

TOE TOUCH

Here is a little by little method for performing a toe contact for seniors:

1.Start with the useful resource of repute right now along side your ft collectively and palms at your elements.

2.Inhale and raise your hands up in the direction of the ceiling.

three.Exhale and slowly bend ahead at the waist, accomplishing your fingers towards your toes.

four.Try to touch your toes or as far down as you could simply reach.

five.Hold this role for a few seconds even as respiration deeply.

6.Slowly upward push once more as much as a status function at the equal time as inhaling.

7.Repeat this workout for a complete of 10 repetitions.

Remember to pay interest for your body and best skip as a ways as you revel in cushty. It's critical to keep correct posture in the direction of the workout and avoid jerky movements.

CAT-COW STRETCH

To do the cat-cow stretch for seniors grade by grade:

1.Start on your palms and knees, collectively along with your wrists straight away underneath your shoulders and your knees immediately under your hips.

2.Inhale and arch your lower back, lifting your head and tailbone in the direction of the ceiling.

three.Exhale and round your spine, tucking your chin in your chest and bringing your tailbone towards your knees.

4.Repeat the collection, inhaling into the cow pose and exhaling into the cat pose.

5.Move at a comfortable tempo and attention on synchronizing your breath along side your moves.

6.Do 10-15 repetitions, or as many as feels comfortable on your body.

STANDING CALF STRETCH

Here is a step-via-step method for acting popularity calf stretches for seniors:

1.Stand dealing with a wall collectively collectively with your hands on the wall at shoulder top.

2.Step decrease again in conjunction with your right foot, maintaining your heel at the ground, and bend your left knee slightly.

3.Lean forward, pressing your arms into the wall, till you experience a stretch in your proper calf.

four.Hold the placement for 15-30 seconds, then lighten up.

five.Repeat the stretch at the alternative facet.

Be positive to breathe deeply as you stretch and save you if you sense any ache.

STANDING ANKLE STRETCH

Here is a step-thru-step method for performing the reputation ankle stretch for seniors:

1.Stand up proper away with your feet shoulder-width apart.

2.Step ahead together with your left foot at the same time as retaining your right foot flat on the floor.

three.Bend your left knee whilst keeping a right now posture. Keep your proper leg immediately.

4.Gently press your left knee beforehand at the same time as retaining your heel at the ground.

five.Hold the place for approximately 15 to 30 seconds, relying on your consolation diploma.

6.Release the pressure and go again to your starting function.

7.Switch legs and repeat the gadget together with your right foot.

CHILD'S POSE

To perform Child's pose stretch for seniors, have a look at the ones steps:

1.Begin in your palms and knees on an workout mat or carpet.

2.Sit decrease again onto your heels and stretch your arms out in the the front of you.

three.Keep your fingers at shoulder distance aside and your fingers at the floor.

four.Slowly tuck your chin and lean ahead, stretching your complete body.

five.Hold this function for 30 seconds to a minute.

6.Release the stretch via slowly bobbing up to a seated characteristic.

SPHINX POSE

To perform the Sphinx pose stretch for seniors, follow the ones step by step instructions:

1.Begin thru mendacity flat on your belly together along side your forearms on the ground, elbows immediately beneath your shoulders.

2.Engage your center and raise your torso off the ground, keeping your forearms and elbows pressed into the ground.

3.Hold the pose for 20-30 seconds, taking deep breaths.

four.Lower your body back off to the beginning feature and repeat the pose as a great deal as five instances.

five.Remember to concentrate in your body and now not push your self too an extended way beyond your person comfort stage.

SPINAL TWIST

Here is a step by step device for doing the spinal twist stretch for seniors:

1.Start with the resource of sitting on a mat or cushty surface.

2.Cross your proper leg over your left knee, placing your right foot at the floor.

three.Slowly twist your torso to the right, setting your left elbow at the outside of your proper knee.

four.Hold the stretch for 10-15 seconds, feeling the stretch thru your once more and center.

5.Release the stretch and transfer sides, crossing your left leg over your right knee and twisting to the left.

6.Repeat the stretch on every aspects numerous instances in advance than reputation up.

PIGEON POSE

Here is a grade by grade approach for Pigeon pose stretch for seniors:

1.Begin on all fours with your fingers and knees on the floor in table-pinnacle position.

2.Slide your right knee in advance inside the route of your proper hand. Position your proper ankle near your left wrist.

three.Stretch your left leg all over again, straightening your knee and aligning your thigh to the ground.

four.Slowly skip your right foot to the left aspect of your mat so that your proper shin is angled in the the front of your left hip.

5.Keep your hips squared to the the the the front of your mat.

6.Stretch your fingers ahead, grounding your elbows and forearms to the ground.

7.Relax your torso onto the right thigh.

8.Breathe deeply and maintain for numerous deep breaths.

9.To launch, gently press your fingers into the floor and shift your weight again to desk-pinnacle feature.

10.Repeat on the opposite factor.

SEATED EAGLE POSE

Step thru the use of step device for Seated Eagle Pose stretch for seniors:

1.Sit up proper now on a chair or mat.

2.Place your ft flat on the floor, hip-width aside.

Chapter 9: Standing Forward Bend

To carry out a standing ahead bend for seniors, take a look at the ones steps:

1. Begin in a status function together with your ft hip-width apart.

2. Inhale and lift your hands above your head.

three. Exhale and hinge ahead from the hips, keeping your spine instantly and accomplishing your fingertips toward the ground.

4. If you are not capable of attain the ground, region your fingers for your thighs and bend your knees barely.

five. Hold the pose for severa breaths, then inhale and slowly come returned as a good deal as fame.

6. Repeat as preferred.

Always cope with your body and do now not push your self past your limits. If you have got were given were given any concerns about whether or now not this pose is suitable for you, talk with a licensed yoga trainer or healthcare practitioner.

WARRIOR II POSE

To perform the Warrior II pose stretch for seniors, look at the ones step-through-step commands:

1.Begin in a status function, collectively with your ft hip-width aside and your fingers at your sides.

2.Step your left foot decrease again, in order that your ft are without a doubt about 3-4 ft aside. Keep each ft facing earlier.

three.Turn your left foot in order that it's far at a forty five-degree attitude. Your right foot want to even though be going thru earlier.

4.Bring your hands as a first rate deal as shoulder peak, parallel to the floor, along side your palms going through down.

five.While inhaling, bend your right knee so that it's miles at once over your right ankle. Keep your left leg proper away.

6.Exhale and amplify your palms out to the sides, preserving them parallel to the floor. Look ahead over your proper hand.

7.Hold the pose for five-10 breaths, then launch and repeat on the other facet.

Make certain to take note of your body and save you if you revel in any ache or ache. It's commonly an super concept to visit a healthcare professional in advance than beginning a present day workout recurring.

WARRIOR III POSE

Here is a step-by using way of-step method for performing the Warrior III pose stretch for seniors:

1.Begin with the beneficial resource of recognition without delay together along with your feet hip-width apart.

2.Slowly shift your weight onto your left foot.

three.While retaining balance, increase your right foot off the floor and increase it within the lower back of you.

4.At the same time, enlarge your fingers out within the the front of you.

5.Try to preserve a right away line from your fingertips to your ft.

6.Hold the pose for 5-10 deep breaths.

7.Slowly lower your raised leg and palms down to the start characteristic.

8.Repeat the same manner at the opportunity element.

Remember to transport slow and attention on your balance. If you feel lightheaded or dizzy, come out of the pose slowly and take a ruin. Always are seeking advice from a doctor in advance than starting any new exercising habitual.

MOUNTAIN POSE

1.Begin via standing tall in conjunction with your ft shoulder-width aside.

2.Inhale deeply, raising your fingers slowly toward the ceiling.

3.Interlace your fingers above your head, in conjunction with your index arms pointing straight away up.

four.Exhale and slowly bend beforehand from the hips, keeping your again and fingers right now.

five.Let your head and neck loosen up.

6.Hold the pose for some breaths, then inhale and slowly straighten up, raising your arms above your head all yet again.

7.Exhale and decrease your arms for your factors.

DOWNWARD DOG WITH BLOCK

Step thru step way for downward dog with block stretch for seniors:

1.Start in your fingers and knees in a tabletop characteristic, together with your wrists aligned right away underneath your shoulders and your knees without delay below your hips.

2.Place a yoga block at the pinnacle of your mat and step every foot on both thing of the block.

3.Slowly carry your hips up and once more, straightening your legs and arms to go back returned into downward canine pose.

4.Walk your fingers within the course of the decrease lower back of the mat, retaining your feet firmly planted and your knees barely bent.

five.As you exhale, reach for the block with one hand and location it on the lowest pinnacle putting. Inhale and attain for the other block and vicinity it at the identical placing.

6.Take a deep breath in and as you exhale, gently place your palms at the blocks, maintaining your arms at once. This will allow you to hold length on your spine.

7.Keeping your legs straight and your toes firmly planted at the floor, lightly push your hips decrease again toward your heels.

8.Hold this pose for five-10 deep breaths.

9.When you are organized to pop out of the pose, supply your arms once more to the mat and walk your ft toward your palms.

10. Roll as an awful lot as popularity function.

HALF MOON POSE

Step with the beneficial useful resource of step way for Half moon pose stretch for seniors:

1.Begin in a status function and region your proper hand on your hip.

2.Slowly increase your left arm within the route of the sky, keeping it close to your ear.

3.Take a jump forward together with your left foot, turning it barely outward.

four.Lean your frame weight onto your left foot, bending your left knee.

five.Take your right hand off your hip and obtain it in the direction of the ground.

6.Straighten your left knee and raise your proper leg, extending it in the back of you.

7.Stretch your right arm closer to the sky and interest your gaze on your left hand.

8.Hold for severa deep breaths, then lightly release and transfer aspects.

SEATED MOUNTAIN POSE

For this seated mountain pose stretch, you will want to:

1.Sit tall and straight away on a chair with every ft on the floor

2.Hold onto the edges of the chair alongside aspect your hands

3.Inhale deeply

four.Exhale slowly

Chapter 10: Boat Pose

To carry out the boat pose stretch for seniors, follow the little by little method below:

1.Begin thru sitting on a mat or cushty floor together with your legs stretched out inside the the front of you.

2.Slowly bend your knees and raise your toes off the ground, bringing your shins parallel to the ground.

3.Extend your palms without delay out within the the front of you at shoulder diploma.

four.Hold this position for 10-30 seconds, step by step growing the period as you turn out to be greater cushty with the pose.

five.Release the pose thru lowering your ft to the ground and returning to a seated feature.

GARLAND POSE

Here is a step by step approach for the Garland pose stretch for seniors:

1.Start with the aid of fame along side your toes barely wider than hip distance.

2.Turn your toes out to a snug angle.

3.Bend your knees and lower your hips inside the route of the floor.

4.Bring your arms collectively in the front of your chest in a prayer function.

five.Use your elbows to softly press your knees open.

6.Hold this pose for severa breaths, keeping your lower decrease returned at once and your chest lifted.

7.Slowly release the pose and stand all over again as much as beginning feature.

BIG TOE POSE

To perform the huge toe pose stretch for seniors, observe those steps:

1.Begin in a seated characteristic alongside side your legs extended out within the the front of you.

2.Bend your proper knee and vicinity the only of your proper foot on your left inner thigh.

3.Take hold of your right big toe collectively along with your right hand.

four.Inhale and raise your left arm right away up.

5.Exhale and begin to fold ahead over your left leg.

6.Pull gently to your big toe to deepen the stretch within the once more of your leg.

7.Hold for five-10 deep breaths.

eight.Slowly come up and launch your foot.

nine.Repeat on the opposite aspect.

HALF LORD OF THE FISHES POSE

Half lord of the fishes pose is a seated twist pose this is extremely good for stretching the hips, backbone and shoulders. Here are the step-with the beneficial resource of-step commands for seniors to carry out this pose:

1.Sit on the ground together collectively along with your legs out in the the front of you, then bend your knees and slide your left foot beneath your right leg to the outside of your proper hip. Your left foot want to be flat at the floor.

2.Bring your right foot over your left knee and place it at the floor.

three.Place your right hand in the lower returned of your decrease again and press down onto the ground to assist boom the backbone.

4.Inhale and raise your left arm in the course of the ceiling.

five.Exhale and twist your torso to the right while placing your left elbow at the out of doors of your right knee.

6.Continue to press your right hand down into the ground to growth your backbone and deepen the twist.

7.Hold this pose for 30 seconds to at least one minute, then release and transfer aspects.

COOL DOWN

Many people are unaware of the importance of relax in stretching. Cool down is a period of slight exercise after excessive or extended pastime. The most common kind of cool down is on foot, however it is able to moreover include some different bodily interest which include jogging, cycling, or swimming. Cool down enables to little by little deliver your coronary coronary heart rate and breathing again to everyday tiers which dispose of lactic acid and different byproducts from the muscle corporations. This lets in for blood go along with the float, oxygen delivery, and distinct nutrients to return again into contact with the muscle tissues cells once more. It's essential which you do that because you do now not want your frame to enjoy unexpected changes in temperature after running out that could reason damage. It's excellent to generally begin with a mild loosen up and then development to strolling or strolling.

The relax is the sluggish lower intensive at the prevent of your exercising. This can be completed with the beneficial aid of sincerely performing bodily games which is probably loads less intense than on the begin of your exercise session. The purpose of cooling down is to allow your coronary coronary heart fee, respiration, and frame temperature to head returned to normal ranges. Stretching after a fab down facilitates prevent harm through loosening tight muscle mass and tendons and additionally reduces soreness following workout. Cooling down also allows blood vessels near the pores and skin's surface to contract, on the way to decrease pores and skin temperature.

How do I properly do calm down?

You need to start your calm down session through the usage of shifting your frame slowly and through the usage of taking prolonged, deep breathes. Then you could begin taking walks or walking at an easy pace. You have to hold taking walks or jogging for approximately five minutes after which take a few different spoil for about three minutes. Then you need to regularly growth the amount of time you're taking walks or on foot till you are finished. Your goal is to surrender with a entire of about 15-20 mins of mild bodily interest on the prevent of your workout consultation.

When should I do my loosen up?

It's first-class to do your relax after workout as it lets in your body to regularly dispose of lactic acid and special byproducts that have been produced at some stage in your workout. It moreover enables supply your coronary heart price, respiratory, and blood glide lower back to ordinary degrees. You can do a groovy down at the cease of each workout consultation or in case you're doing more than one in a day. That manner, you could assist aid your muscular tissues whilst even though allowing them proper healing time.

When should not I do my relax?

You need to not do a fab down in case you are so worn-out which you are unable to finish it nicely. If you're so tired that it takes you longer than a couple of minutes to walk or jog, then maintain exercise until your coronary coronary heart price and breathing cross again to ordinary degrees. Otherwise, in case you sincerely stand spherical for a few minutes and do nothing till you sense extra comfortable, then you definately won't be properly recovering from your exercise.

What else ought to I understand?

Always stretch lightly and slowly following a cool down that permits you to save you damage. If it's miles hard for you to walk or jog for 15-20 minutes after your exercise, then growth the time often over time because it will become much much less complex. You moreover need to keep away from stretching proper after operating out because of the fact this is whilst your muscle businesses are at their warmest. It's additionally higher if you keep away from doing sports activities activities consisting of taking walks or biking proper after your workout because of the reality you may not need to move very slowly at the same time as doing all of your relax because of fatigue.

SAFETY PRECAUTIONS

You're possibly used to seeing articles on your social media feed approximately fitness developments, however did you apprehend that seniors have some of unique health complications? As we age, our muscle mass end up weaker and lots much less bendy. That's why it is critical for seniors to exercising regularly, whether or not it is through yoga or weightlifting. The maximum important detail is to start out sluggish. It's now not uncommon for older adults to grow to be with muscle strains and sprains with unsuitable stretching techniques. It may be a first-rate concept for seniors to take an exercise class or hire a professional fitness instructor to help with stretching sports activities.

When appearing stretches, it's far important to have the proper posture and alignment to your body earlier than beginning. Otherwise, you hazard injuring your self even similarly. You need to make certain which you're inhaling deeply thru your nostril and out through your mouth for optimum impact in some unspecified time in the future of the stretches.

Everyone can benefit from stretching, however it is specially crucial for seniors. Who knew it is able to be so unstable? Keep studying to discover how you may make certain your dad and mom are strong once they stretch.

If you've got got cherished ones which can be seniors, possibilities are they may have fallen prey to an damage and want clinical hobby. Some of the most not unusual injuries for this group of people encompass muscle tears and tendon ruptures, which might be most customarily because of stretching sporting activities completed incorrectly or too aggressively.

Get your circle of relatives to have a laugh on the same time as they workout through making sure they do the right stretches and the use of the right materials! Here are a few suggestions to help you prevent injuries from taking area:

1.Make high-quality you operate the right materials.

The first maximum critical trouble you can do is ensure you use the proper substances for his or her stretching sporting sports. To be at the steady factor, continuously pass for better quality immoderate-everyday general overall performance rubber, which can be quite high priced but is a lot extra stable than different substances like NBR or latex. Look for superb elastomer made with herbal rubber in location of synthetics — the ones have hundreds higher elasticity and tear resistance, so they're manner greater durable common.

2.Practice proper shape.

Another issue you should be careful for is your loved one's form whilst they will be exercise. Stretching is a important part of brushing and flossing teeth, but a whole lot of seniors do it the incorrect way. Even for diabetics, stretching bodily video games should be executed nicely and that they must exceptional stretch muscular tissues at the beginning and result in their day to maintain their tendons sturdy and healthful; otherwise, you may harm them — relying on how bendy they're, they may emerge as with tendon ruptures or muscle tears. Watch them carefully as they stretch body factors like their hamstrings or quadriceps, further to their yet again. Sometimes, seniors will overextend positive joints, which could purpose pretty a bit of pain and pain.

Chapter 11: Things To Consider

You want to first accomplish the ones devices so you can put together for starting a stretching utility. Even at the same time as it is able to seem easy to start stretching frequently, there may be a drastically better chance of damage if you are not well organized. In order to test this system you selected, education can even assist you recognise exactly what you have got emerge as engaged in.

Consult Your Doctor

The maximum important issue you could do earlier than starting a stretching utility is to talk approximately your current health together with your medical scientific doctor. They is probably capable of recommend you at the areas you want to popularity on and the manner regularly you have to stretch to enhance your health. They may also additionally prescribe you nutrients or drugs when you have coronary coronary coronary heart or bone issues.

Find a Trainer

You will want to discover a trainer in case you are new to stretching or in case your physician indicates that you art work with someone to hobby on high quality issues. You may additionally moreover attend publications or discover a person via your close by fitness center if you want help stretching. However, you may want to look a physiotherapist to help you when you have physical limitations.

Locate a Location

Finding an opening in which you could do your stretching sporting sports maximum correctly and with out issue is endorsed. You would possibly probably determine to do this at home, the gymnasium, or the community center in your place. You'll want to make certain you continuously have get right of entry to to these gadgets because of the fact that wonderful stretches call for additonal system. Numerous network centers will provide little fitness regions which are exceptional for running out, and they are regularly a ways less luxurious than gyms.

Dress as it should be

You can stretch lots less difficult in case you put on the right clothing, however it might not have to be something fancy or expensive, so do no longer strain. You need to get wearing a few difficulty that won't in any way limit your movements. This can be spandex or unique form-turning into clothing, like yoga pants.

Buy Some Stretching Equipment

You can do pretty a few stretches without any specific device, however having a few simple gadget can make sure stretches extra stable and plenty less complex for your developing vintage body. Stretch or resistance bands artwork wonders for simplifying and improving the effectiveness of many stretches. A yoga mat is good for cushioning your frame on the equal time as finishing any stretches from the ground, and an incline board offers you an inclined floor for multiple leg stretches.

There also are numerous gadget designed especially for stretching. These are a remarkable approach to start started out because they encourage you to do the stretch efficaciously, which permits you prevent damage and could growth the stretch's efficacy. Unfortunately, they are generally as an alternative highly-priced, therefore it is commonly lots fundamental if you may find out a gym that offers them.

The most effective thing left to do is maintain reading to observe more about stretching so that you can begin stretching each day after you've got were given had been given everything equipped.

Chapter 12: Significance Of Stretching For Seniors

Stretching holds an extensive significance for seniors, mainly those matured 60 or extra. As the frame is going thru regular changes with age, integrating ordinary stretching into one's fashionable becomes useful in addition to crucial.

Here is an extensive investigation of the significance of Stretching for seniors:

Further advanced Adaptability and Scope of Movement: Maturing frequently turns on a slow decrease in joint adaptability and muscle flexibility. Normal Stretching neutralizes this decay via advancing joint oil, which upgrades portability and continues a complete scope of movement. Seniors who stretch revel in prolonged ease in appearing regular wearing activities and are plenty less willing to firmness.

Upgraded Flow: Stretching increments blood movement to the muscle tissues, advancing talented go along with the drift. Further evolved dissemination benefits seniors thru conveying oxygen and dietary dietary supplements to the muscles and organs, assisting with cell repair and via and huge essentialness.

Diminished Muscle Pressure and Agony: Solid stress and inconvenience can raise with age, prompting troubles like back struggling and firmness. Stretching mitigates muscle strain, handing over advanced pressure and diminishing the chance of constant torment. Seniors who integrate today's extending into their ordinary often file encountering lots a great deal less uneasiness.

Further advanced Stance: Age-associated changes in bone thickness and muscle energy will have an impact on pose. Stretching practices that focus on center muscle tissues and the backbone add to all of the much more likely stance, which consequently can prompt advanced respiration, reduced burden at the frame, and a more young appearance.

Injury Avoidance: Seniors are extra helpless to falls and wounds due to reduced bone thickness and muscle energy. Stretching similarly develops equilibrium, soundness, and coordination. By enhancing those viewpoints, seniors can decrease their gamble of falls and ensuing wounds.

Joint Wellbeing: Stretching allows with preserving up with the steadiness of joints thru saving their regular grease and forestalling solidness. It likewise lessens the gamble of creating degenerative joint conditions, for instance, joint pain, which may be in particular large for seniors.

Stress Alleviation and Mental Prosperity: Taking element in Stretching practices advances unwinding thru manner of turning in endorphins — the body's ordinary "lighthearted" chemical compounds. This provides to decreased emotions of hysteria, in addition advanced kingdom of thoughts, and better intellectual prosperity.

Better Rest: Seniors frequently struggle with relaxation problems. Stretching, especially as a detail of a quieting sleep time time desk, can help with loosening up the body and brain, prompting further superior rest wonderful.

Keeping up with Autonomy: Safeguarding actual functionality is vital for seniors' autonomy. By integrating ordinary Stretching into their normal exercise, seniors can hold up with their capability to carry out normal assignments, lessening dependence on assist from others.

Social Commitment: Bunch Stretching conferences or training provide seniors a valuable threat to companion and interface with buddies, encouraging a experience of nearby location and having an area that emphatically impacts intellectual and profound fitness.

Positive Taking care of oneself Custom: Stretching isn't always pretty a lot real benefits; a careful workout advances searching after oneself and mindfulness. Seniors who popularity on a fashionable Stretching ordinary are putting sources into their own prosperity, cultivating a high pleasant courting with their our bodies.

Generally, Stretching for seniors rises above the real place. It's a whole manner to address keeping a super of life, advancing freedom, and helping highbrow and profound prosperity.

By embracing the act of Stretching, seniors can embody the years earlier with a greater noteworthy feeling of imperative, solace, and satisfaction.

Benefits of Regular Stretching

Further advanced Adaptability and Scope of Movement: Normal Stretching enables seniors maintain up with or perhaps beautify their adaptability, empowering them to transport all the extra uninhibitedly and without problems. This turns into critical for everyday wearing activities, upgrading their popular private delight.

Improved Joint Wellbeing: Stretching advances the power of joints with the useful resource of growing synovial liquid introduction, which greases up the joints and diminishes the gamble of firmness or inconvenience. This is especially big in maintaining up with versatility as seniors age.

Decreased Muscle Pressure and Torment: Extending loosens up muscular tissues, turning in strain that may set off struggling and misery. Seniors can encounter remedy from steady muscle snugness or inflammation, which includes to a better feeling of prosperity.

Further advanced Stance: Stretching practices specializing in middle muscle mass and the backbone can upload to more without problems act. This assists seniors with reputation taller similarly to helps their lower back health and stops the development of unfortunate stance associated issues.

Upgraded Equilibrium and Coordination: Stretching schedules that consolidate balance practices further boom soundness and coordination, lessening the gamble of falls and wounds that can be specially demanding for seniors.

Decreased Hazard of Injury: Less wounds can arise at the same time as muscular tissues and joints are adaptable. By routinely charming in extending, seniors can restriction the gamble of lines, hyper-extends, and one-of-a-kind wounds, empowering them to live dynamic and unfastened.

Better Blood Course: Stretching improvements blood flow into to muscle businesses and tissues, advancing inexperienced drift. Further advanced blood glide upholds cellular well-being, allows with tissue restoration, and provides to typically cardiovascular prosperity.

Stress Alleviation and Unwinding: Stretching triggers the appearance of endorphins, everyday "happy skip lucky" chemical compounds that fortify unwinding and reduce stress. Seniors can appreciate worked on intellectual prosperity and a more inspirational angle on lifestyles.

Further evolved Rest Quality: Integrating Stretching proper right into a everyday time table can prompt higher rest. The unwinding setting out impacts of Stretching upload to more peaceful evenings, permitting seniors to awaken feeling revived.

Better Assimilation: Some Stretching postures can animate the stomach related framework, advancing better absorption and reducing everyday belly associated inconveniences which could have an effect on seniors.

Positive Brain Body Association: Ordinary Stretching empowers care and a more grounded affiliation between the frame and psyche. Seniors can foster a extra notable interest of their frame's necessities, advancing searching after oneself and whole fitness.

Social Commitment: Taking detail in bunch extending conferences can domesticate a experience of fellowship among seniors. This social perspective gives to intellectual prosperity and battles sensations of seclusion.

Keeping up with Autonomy: By enhancing adaptability, equilibrium, and typically actual capability, seniors can preserve up with their autonomy and maintain on acting ordinary wearing activities without relying intensely on help.

Long haul Health: Integrating everyday Stretching right right into a senior's standard is an interest in prolonged haul fitness. Seniors who interest on Stretching are effective to stumble upon a extra incredible of existence as they age.

Chapter 13: Basic Stretching Guidelines

Warm-Up Techniques:

Prior to leaping into stretches, heating up the body is essential for increment blood flow into, improve the inner warm temperature stage's, and get geared up muscle mass for more brilliant development. Warm-up carrying sports activities may additionally moreover need to incorporate touchy on foot, arm swings, or taking walks set up. This diminishes the gamble of injury and improves the viability of the stretching time desk.

Breathing and Unwinding Methods:

Careful respiration is important to successful stretching. Profound and musical respiratory advances unwinding, diminishes strain, and upgrades the frame's adaptability. Breathing in profoundly in advance than a stretch and respiration out as you slip into it could assist muscular tissues unwind and enlarge all the greater effectively.

Appropriate Clothing and Footwear:

Wearing open to get dressed that lets in a complete scope of motion is pivotal. Appropriate shoes, like regular shoes, gives stability and padding, that is in particular fantastic for stability works out. Proper apparel ensures that the frame is not constrained and might flow openly at some stage in stretching.

Hold and Delivery Method:

As you stretch, tenderly straightforwardness into the scenario until you experience a terrific strain. Hold the stretch for 15-30 seconds, allowing the muscle corporations to unwind and extend. Try not to bop or yanking moves because of the truth they're able to harm. Center spherical a sluggish arrival of pressure at the same time as keeping up with everyday enjoyable.

No Aggravation, No Strain:

Seniors should never come across torment on the equal time as stretching.

Inconvenience is excellent, mainly on the same time as looking to further increase adaptability, however sharp or excessive ache indicates that the stretch is excessively forceful and have to be halted proper away.

Stretching ought to be a sensitive and non-stop cycle that regards as some distance as viable.

Integrating Stretching into Day to day Exercises.

Integrating Stretching into everyday carrying occasions turns into an smooth exercise with large blessings for seniors greater than 60, as featured in "Stretching Exercises for Seniors over 60."

Via flawlessly meshing Stretches into regular schedules, humans can improve their adaptability and usually prosperity. Basic behaves like going after a element on a rack, pausing for a minute to stretch after waking, or consolidating Stretches at the same time as sitting inside the the front of the television may want to have an extremely good effect. By incorporating Stretches into every day lifestyles, seniors can continuously construct their scope of movement, lower muscle strain, and enhance joint health. This approach encourages a possible responsibility to looking after oneself, as Stretching will become an innate piece of the day in location of a disengaged task.

With the ones open strategies, the ebook engages seniors to move away on an tour of further superior solace, portability, and a reestablished zing for everyday dwelling.

Chapter 14: Upper Body Stretches

Neck and Shoulder Stretches:

Tenderly slant your head aside, bringing your ear inside the path of your shoulder.

Utilize your hand to direct the stretch, keeping for 15-30 seconds on each side.

For shoulder Stretches, roll your shoulders in reverse and ahead to assuage stress.

Arm and Wrist Stretches:

Broaden one arm without delay earlier than you, fingers going through up.

Utilize the alternative hand to delicately pull the palms over again, Stretching the lower arm and wrist.

Hold for 15-30 seconds on every aspect to improve wrist adaptability.

Chest Opener Stretch:

Fasten your palms at the back of your lower once more, tenderly lifting your hands out of your body to open up the chest.

Hold for 15-30 seconds. This stretch further develops pose and balances slumping.

Shoulder Bone Press:

Sit or stand tall and delicately press your shoulder bones together, feeling a stretch at some point of your chest.

Hold for more than one moments and shipping.

This stretch works on higher decrease back strength and stance.

Rear arm muscle companies Stretch:

Arrive at one arm above and curve the elbow, permitting your hand to drop down your decrease again.

To push at the bowed elbow, make use of the opposite hand delicately.

Hold for 15-30 seconds on every side to Stretch the rear arm muscular tissues.

Wrist Flexor and Extensor Stretches:

Broaden one arm earlier than you together with your palm searching up (flexor stretch) and later on down (extensor stretch).

Tenderly shy away to your hands at the side of your opposite hand to Stretch the wrist and reduce arm.

Hold for 15-30 seconds on each aspect.

Upper Back Stretch:

Driving your palms away, grip your fingers in advance than you while adjusting your higher lower again.

Feel a stretch amongst your shoulder bones.

Hold for 15-30 seconds to ease pinnacle another time strain.

Side Arm Stretch:

Broaden one arm above and curve it at the elbow, arriving at your hand toward the opposite element.

Tenderly push on the elbow along with your opposite hand to boom the stretch.

Hold for 15-30 seconds on every factor.

Lower arm Stretch:

One arm ought to be stretched out in advance than you, palm down.

Utilize your contrary hand to delicately pull lower returned on your hands, extending the decrease arm muscle corporations.

Hold for 15-30 seconds on every aspect.

Finger and Hand Stretch:

Entwine your fingers and stretch your fingers beforehand, hands confronting far from you.

Hold for 15-30 seconds to growth your fingers and arms, advancing adaptability and solace.

Chapter 15: Lower Body Stretches

Leg and Hip Stretches:

Sit or rests in your again.

Delicately bring one knee inside the path of your chest, preserving inside the lower back of the thigh.

Feel a stretch on your hip and thigh.

Hold for 15-30 seconds on each factor to artwork on hip adaptability.

Quad Stretch:

Stand close to an extended lasting help.

Twist one knee and tenderly grasp your decrease leg at the back of you, pulling your heel in the direction of your bum.

Hold for 15-30 seconds on each issue to stretch the front of your thigh.

Hamstring Stretch:

Sit on the threshold of a seat.

Set one leg at the right song out in advance than you with the heel down.

Pivot at your hips to incline quite earlier, feeling a stretch in the direction of the rear of your thigh.

Hold for 15-30 seconds on every side.

Internal Thigh Stretch:

Sit on the floor and produce the bottoms of your ft collectively, permitting your knees to drop out to the edges.

Feel a stretch as you delicately press your elbows closer to your internal thighs.

Hold for 15-30 seconds to similarly boom inward thigh adaptability.

Calf Stretch:

Put your fingers at the wall whilst you stand confronting it.

Keep your foot proper away as you make a stride lower back.

Incline forward, twisting the the the front knee, and experience a stretch in the calf of the lower returned leg.

Hold for 15-30 seconds on every issue.

Lower leg Circles:

Sit in an agreeable function.

Lift one foot off the ground and tenderly flip your lower leg in clockwise and afterward counterclockwise circles.

This keeps up with lower leg versatility and decreases solidness.

Toe Flexor Stretch:

Place one lower leg over the knee of the opportunity at the equal time as sitting on a seat.

Tenderly press down at the crossed leg's toes, feeling a stretch in the foot's top.

Hold for 15-30 seconds on each aspect.

Achilles Ligament Stretch:

Stand confronting a wall, hands on it for assist.

Stage one foot once more, keeping it right now.

Twist the the front knee and incline beforehand, feeling a stretch within the over again decrease leg.

Hold for 15-30 seconds on each difficulty.

Heel Line Stretch:

Sit on the brink of a seat.

Broaden one leg without delay earlier than you and flex your foot, arching your foot in the direction of the roof.

Feel a stretch to your calf.

Hold for 15-30 seconds on every issue.

Foot Back rub with Tennis Ball:

Place a tennis ball beneath one foot as you plunk down.

Turn your foot over the ball, using sensitive anxiety.

This eases strain and distress in the foot.

Integrating the ones lower frame Stretch into an everyday ordinary can growth advanced decrease frame adaptability, equilibrium, and solace for seniors north of 60. Continuously focus on safety and be privy to your body even as gambling out those stretches.

Chapter 16: Core And Back Stretches

Delicate Back Stretch:

Lie on your all over again with knees bowed.

Tenderly include your knees to your chest, feeling a stretch to your lower again.

Hold for 15-30 seconds to mitigate strain and increase spinal adaptability.

Feline Cow Stretch:

Get on all fours.

Curve your decrease lower returned vertical (like a feline) even as respiratory out, then, at that factor, drop your belly toward the ground (like a cow) whilst inhaling.

This stretch advances portability and unwinding of the backbone.

Youngster's Posture:

Bow down and recline onto your heels.

Arrive at your hands earlier, bringing your chest all the way down to the ground.

This stretch delicately extends and ensures pressure inside the lower again

Situated Spinal Curve:

Sit on a seat or the floor with legs extended.

Delicately turn your middle toward the had been given leg while getting one leg over the other.

To expand the stretch, rent the hand inverse your very non-public.

Hold for 15-30 seconds on each facet.

Pelvic Slant:

Lie to your lower again with knees twisted.

Tenderly press your lower another time into the floor, then curve it faraway from the floor, moving your pelvis.

This stretch attracts in and discharge the muscles of the decrease again.

Span Posture:

Knees bowed and feet stage, lie to your back. By raising your hips over the floor, form an extension collectively along with your body.

This stretch actuates the lower another time and draws within the center muscle businesses.

Spinal Expansion Stretch:

Sit on a seat with a immediately decrease decrease back.

Put your fingers to your lower decrease returned and tenderly recline, curving your backbone.

Hold for a fast period, then reset your body to the start characteristic.

This stretch advances lower lower back adaptability.

Side Curve Stretch:

Sit or stand tall and arrive at one arm above.

Tenderly curve your middle aside, feeling a stretch alongside the opposite element.

Hold for 15-30 seconds on each issue to Stretch the slanted muscle businesses.

Quadruped Arm and Leg Raise:

Get on all fours.

Expand one arm in advance and the opposite leg in contrary, keeping up with stability.

This stretch attracts within the center muscular tissues whilst advancing balance and equilibrium.

Hip Flexor Stretch with Side Lean:

Bow on one knee and increase the opportunity leg earlier than you.

Delicately lean your center apart, feeling a stretch within the hip flexors and obliques.

Hold for 15-30 seconds on every facet.

Chapter 17: Balance And Flexibility Exercises

Standing Equilibrium Exercises:

Stand close to a stable floor for help.

Lift one foot off the floor and equilibrium on the other foot.

Hold for 15-30 seconds, then, at that element, transfer elements.

This workout further develops equilibrium and stability in the decrease body.

Heel-Toe Walk:

Make slow strides, placing the effect detail of one foot straightforwardly earlier than the feet of the alternative foot.

This troubles stability and further develops stroll coordination.

Seat Yoga Stances:

Take component in located yoga represents that emphasis on balance, as an instance, lifting every leg in turn or rehearsing situated tree present.

These postures similarly increase stability on the equal time as providing the help of a seat.

Adaptability Schedule:

Play out a succession of stretches specializing in one-of-a-type muscle gatherings, preserving each stretch for 15-30 seconds.

Incorporate stretches for the legs, hips, fingers, and shoulders to boom by way of using the use of and massive adaptability.

Kendo Developments:

Practice slow and recollect Judo tendencies that increase equilibrium, coordination, and flexibility.

The streaming actions enhance physical and highbrow prosperity.

Leg Swings:

Clutch a assist and delicately swing one leg in advance and in opposite.

This effective interest similarly develops leg adaptability and equilibrium.

Lower leg Letters in order:

While positioned, bring one foot off the ground and "kingdom" the letters in order in the air making use of your foot.

This workout further develops lower leg versatility and solidness.

Single-Leg Deadlift:

Stand on one leg at the identical time as often pivoting ahead at the hips, growing the alternative leg in the again of you for stability.

This exercising improves hamstring adaptability and equilibrium.

Seat Helped Leg Stretch:

Place one leg out in advance than you even as sitting on a seat.

Utilize your fingers to transport after your ft, feeling a stretch towards the rear of the leg delicately.

Hold for 15-30 seconds on each issue.

Yoga Sun Greetings:

Put your very own twist on the commonplace solar greeting movements.

These streaming traits hook up with the entire frame, enhancing adaptability and equilibrium.

Integrating these equilibrium and flexibility practices proper into a preferred everyday can further broaden power, prevent falls, and improve typically speaking versatility for seniors more than 60. As regular, hobby on health and pick out out practices that in form your solace and capacities.

DAILY STRETCHING ROUTINE

15-Minute Daily Routine

Duration: 20-1/2-hour

Warm-Up (five minutes):

Start with mild cardio motion like on foot installation or walking to increment blood flow into.

Perform delicate neck circles, shoulder rolls, and decrease leg revolutions to installation the frame.

Upper body Stretches (five minutes):

Neck Side Stretch (30 seconds each aspect):

Tenderly slant your head apart, extending your neck muscle groups.

Arm Across Chest Stretch (30 seconds each side):

Expand one arm across your chest, making use of the opposite hand to tenderly press.

Rear arm muscle corporations Stretch (30 seconds every component):

Arrive at one arm above and curve the elbow, making use of the opportunity hand to assist.

Chest Opener Stretch (30 seconds):

Fasten your hands behind your decrease lower back and delicately enhance, organising your chest.

Wrist and Lower arm Stretch (30 seconds every issue):

Expand one arm with the palm up and delicately pull the fingers again.

Center and Back Stretches (five minutes):

Feline Cow Stretch (1 2nd):

Get on all fours, curving your again vertical and descending.

Situated Spinal Contort (30 seconds every element):

Sit with one leg have been given over the alternative and tenderly contort your middle.

Span Posture (30 seconds):

Lie to your decrease lower back, increase your hips off the ground, and connect to your center.

Lower Body Stretches (5 mins):

Quad Stretch (30 seconds every factor):

Stand near a help, twist one knee, and keep your decrease leg inside the again of you.

Hamstring Stretch (30 seconds each issue):

Sit on a seat's side and develop one leg without delay, going after your feet.

Calf Stretch (30 seconds every thing):

Stand confronting a wall, diploma one foot again, and incline earlier to boom the calf.

Equilibrium and Unwinding (5 mins):

Standing Equilibrium Exercise (30 seconds each leg):

Lift one foot off the floor and equilibrium, drawing in your middle.

Breathing and Unwinding (3 mins):

Sit or rests with out troubles, close to your eyes, and practice profound enjoyable.

Breathe in via your nostril, breathe out thru your mouth, and allow pass of stress.

Cool Down (5 minutes):

Perform sensitive complete frame extends like a beforehand crease or positioned hamstring stretch.

End with multiple whole breaths in an agreeable located role.

This a protracted way attaining 20 brief every day ordinary stretching habitual gives a complete way to address improving adaptability, equilibrium, and unwinding for seniors over 60. Adjust the each day workout in your solace stage and do not forget that consistency is critical to encountering the benefits over the lengthy haul.

Chapter 18: Understanding The Aging Body

The Impact of Aging on Mobility and Flexibility

Our our our bodies obviously alternate as we age, which encompass a slow loss of mobility and flexibility. These modifications could have a huge effect on our functionality to carry out day by day obligations, preserve independence, and live an active way of lifestyles. Understanding the impacts of getting older on mobility and flexibility is important for seniors and caregivers to set up appropriate techniques and exercising physical activities to effectively control those problems.

The normal loss of muscle groups and power, referred to as sarcopenia, is one of the key reasons contributing to the deterioration in mobility and versatility with age. Our our our bodies undergo a decline within the quantity and duration of muscle fibers as we age, ensuing in diminished muscular tone and energy. This reduction of muscular tissues impairs our ability to create strain and perform movements, making such things as strolling, hiking stairs, and maintaining stability harder.

Aside from muscle loss, growing old reduces the energy of our joints, tendons, and ligaments. Our our our bodies' connective tissues come to be a great deal less elastic and extra inflexible over time, limiting our variety of motion and generating stiffness. This loss of joint flexibility can reason soreness, decreased motion, and an stepped forward danger of harm.

Other age-associated ailments and variables can boom the impact of getting antique on mobility and versatility. Chronic issues like arthritis, osteoporosis, and joint degeneration can motive joint ache, irritation, and further movement limits. Muscle imbalances and reduced flexibility moreover can be because of horrible posture and sedentary lifestyles.

However, commonplace stretching sports activities can assist lessen the damaging results of developing antique on mobility and versatility. Seniors can advantage an entire lot of blessings with the aid of the usage of using including stretching wearing activities into their every day lives, which encompass improved physical functioning and popular properly-being.

Stretching sports increase muscular flexibility and joint shape of movement, which improves mobility and lowers the risk of falls and injuries. Seniors can prevent the herbal stiffening technique and hold or even growth their potential to do each day activities thru stretching their muscle companies and connective tissues. Flexibility improves stability and coordination via taking into account a greater fluid and herbal stroll.

Stretching physical video games also can assist to lessen muscle tension and promote relaxation. Stretching muscle agencies stimulates blood flow to the tissues, improving oxygen and nutrient availability. This greater great flow into can relieve muscle pain, stiffness, and contribute to a preferred enjoy of nicely-being.

Stretching bodily sports for seniors may moreover have a extraordinary effect on highbrow fitness in addition to bodily advantages. Stretching on a regular basis improves strain reduce charge and rest. Stretching bodily activities can assist seniors hobby on the prevailing 2nd, lessen tension, and increase widespread highbrow clarity thru the usage of setting up a mind-body connection.

Furthermore, stretching on a ordinary basis can enhance posture and alignment, reducing the hazard of developing musculoskeletal ailments along side once more soreness and postural imbalances. Seniors can maintain a greater upright posture, beautify stability, and decrease joint pain thru manner of strengthening and stretching the muscle corporations that resource the spine and maintaining appropriate enough alignment.

Aging's impact on mobility and flexibility is a herbal phenomenon that might prevent elders' functionality to complete every day obligations and decrease their amazing of life. Regular stretching sporting sports, however, can substantially lessen the ones outcomes. Stretching sports activities enhance muscle flexibility, joint type of movement, and posture, so developing mobility, lowering the risk of falling, and provoking higher physical functioning. Furthermore, stretching sports activities decorate intellectual fitness by means of way of the usage of lowering anxiety and upsetting relaxation. Seniors can maintain an lively and large manner of lifestyles prolonged into their golden years via embracing the advantages of stretching carrying activities.

Common Physical Challenges Faced with the useful resource of Seniors

Our our our bodies change as we age, which may additionally additionally create specific bodily boundaries. These problems may also moreover have a energy on our everyday existence, independence, and latest nicely-being. Understanding the not unusual bodily limitations that seniors confront is essential for caregivers, healthcare specialists, and seniors themselves to layout a success techniques and interventions.

1. Reduced Muscle Strength: One of the maximum commonplace physical issues that seniors confront is a loss of muscle power and mass. This age-associated deterioration, known as sarcopenia, can bring about reduced muscle power, making common actions like lifting, wearing, and taking walks upstairs extra difficult. Weak muscle tissue may also moreover furthermore increase the threat of falls and harm.

2. Joint Stiffness and Reduced Flexibility: As we age, our joint mobility and versatility decline. Joints, tendons, and ligaments stiffen and turn out to be tons less elastic, resulting in a restrained type of movement and flexibility. Seniors may additionally have

problem bending, undertaking, or project joint-motion carrying activities. Stiffness can reason ache, suffering, and an prolonged chance of damage.

three. Issues with Balance and Coordination: Balance and coordination are essential for maintaining equilibrium and keeping off falls. However, as they age, many seniors face troubles in these regions. Balance and coordination may be suffering from age-associated modifications within the internal ear, muscle tissue, and sensory perception. This makes it more difficult for elders to pass uneven surfaces, climb stairs, or execute sports activities requiring unique motions.

four. Decreased Cardiovascular Endurance: As we age, our cardiovascular health generally drops. Seniors may have reduced stamina and staying power, making physical interest and retaining an energetic way of lifestyles extra tough. Fatigue, shortness of breath, and boundaries in each day sports can all be signs and symptoms and signs of decreased cardiovascular staying strength.

5. Bone Density Loss: Osteoporosis, described through using lowering bone density and an elevated hazard of fractures, is good sized amongst aged, especially ladies. Even clean falls or incidents can result in fractured bones, posing good sized troubles to mobility and elegant bodily health.

6. Chronic Pain and Inflammation: Many seniors be concerned with the aid of using chronic pain, that is frequently because of age-related troubles such arthritis, osteoarthritis, and degenerative joint sickness. Persistent ache can impair mobility, limit physical hobby, and feature a awful effect on satisfactory of life. Inflammation within the joints and tissues can aggravate these issues, ensuing in stiffness and reduced capability.

7. Vision and Hearing Decline: Aging-associated impairments in imaginative and prescient and listening to can pose physical

troubles for elders. Depth perception, balance, and spatial reputation can all be laid low with decreased seen acuity or taking note of impairment. These problems could make it greater tough for seniors to nicely navigate their environment and take part in sports that depend upon visible or auditory clues.

Slower Reaction Time: As we become older, our reaction time slows down. This has ramifications for sports requiring short reflexes, together with grabbing a falling item or reacting to unexpected conditions. Slower response times can boom the chance of an twist of fate or a fall.

Seniors can gain from masses of interventions and strategies to manipulate these physical troubles. Strength education, balancing sporting events, and versatility workouts can all help decorate muscular energy, joint mobility, and regular bodily feature. A well-balanced and nutritious food regimen, blended with the right dietary nutritional dietary supplements, can help with bone health and customary nicely-being. Canes, walkers, and hearing aids are examples of assistive system which could assist with mobility and compensate for sensory deficiencies. Regular check-u.S.A.With healthcare specialists can useful resource inside the manipulate of persistent illnesses and the renovation of bodily health.

We can improve seniors' extraordinary of life, sell independence, and allow them to age gracefully while preserving physical well-being via spotting and addressing the everyday bodily issues they confront.

Chapter 19: Safety Precautions And Considerations

When performing stretching sporting activities, specially as a senior, it's miles vital to prioritize safety in case you want to avoid accidents and feature a super revel in. You can revel in the blessings of stretching even as keeping off the chance of accidents or strain via following sure smooth protection techniques and problems. Here are a few key hints to endure in thoughts:

1. Consult Your Healthcare practitioner: Before starting any new fitness habitual, talk over with your healthcare practitioner, especially if you have any pre-gift medical ailments or problems. They can offer precise steerage relying on your health scenario and assist you in figuring out which stretching sports are great for you.

2. Preparation Warm up your muscular tissues and joints earlier than beginning any stretching sports. This prepares your body for bodily exercise at the identical time as

moreover reducing your hazard of damage. In order to decorate blood go with the flow and growth your body temperature, include slight motions collectively with taking walks, biking, or marching in location.

3. Begin slowly and step by step. Begin your stretching routine with smooth, slight movements and grade by grade boom the intensity and length through the years. Pushing your self too tough in the starting may additionally harm your muscle groups and joints. Proceed at a snug pace to your body, being attentive to any symptoms of soreness or pain.

4. Focus on Proper Technique: Proper technique is essential for a achievement and steady stretching. Maintain right posture, interact the focused muscle agencies, and use managed motions. Avoid bouncing or jerking motions, which might result in damage. If you're harassed approximately the right technique, consult a professional health

professional or depend on depended on statistics.

five. Respect Your Body's Limits: Everyone's frame is precise, consequently it's miles critical to recognize your very personal. Never skip beyond what's cushty or causes ache at some stage in stretching. Stretching need to revel in like a mild tug or tension in location of abrupt or intense pain. If you sense any ache or discomfort, adapt the interest or are searching out the advice of a healthcare professional.

6. Be Aware of Pre-Existing problems: Be aware about your pointers when you have any pre-current health issues, which consist of arthritis, osteoporosis, or joint problems. Stretches may also want to be modified or avoided absolutely to avoid worsening the ones issues. For advice on appropriate exercises, speak collectively together with your healthcare practitioner or a prepared fitness professional.

7. Use proper Equipment: To enhance safety inside the path of stretching sports activities, use right tool and add-ons. To provide balance and save you falls, don't forget the use of a non-slip exercising mat or rug. Use supportive props which includes chairs or blocks to help with stability or stability within the direction of unique stretches if vital.

8. Stay Hydrated: It's critical to stay hydrated in advance than, all through, and after stretching. Drink water on a everyday basis to live hydrated. Dehydration can impair overall performance and boom the hazard of muscle cramps or dizziness.

nine. Pay Attention to Your Body: During stretching bodily video games, pay unique interest in your frame's indicators. Stop the exercise and get clinical interest when you have any sharp or extended ache, dizziness, shortness of breath, or particular worrying signs and signs and symptoms and signs and signs and symptoms. Your frame is the professional, so constantly be aware of its signs and signs and regulate subsequently.

10. Consistency and Moderation: While consistency is vital for reaping the blessings of stretching sports activities, moderation is also critical. Excessive stretching and repetition can pressure muscle agencies and joints. Aim for normal, balanced stretching practices that offer a modest mission with out setting an excessive amount of stress in your frame.

You can assemble a steady and fun stretching routine that facilitates your popular nicely-being thru following these protection precautions and concerns. Remember to prioritize your fitness and are trying to find expert recommendation as had to offer a customized technique that meets your precise dreams and sports. Stretching ought to be a amusing and exquisite hobby that develops flexibility, mobility, and a better way of life.

Importance of Consulting with a Healthcare Professional

When beginning a stretching exercising ordinary, mainly for seniors, it's miles crucial to emphasize your health and safety. Before beginning any new workout regimen, one of the most crucial moves you could take is to visit a healthcare professional. Here are numerous reasons why consulting with a healthcare expert is important:

1. Individualized Guidance: Healthcare experts have the enjoy and facts to provide individualized steering based definitely really to your character health circumstance, clinical statistics, and specialized wishes, which embody clinical medical doctors, bodily therapists, or exercise physiologists. They can have a take a look at your modern fitness diploma, examine any underlying health problems or injuries, and make suggestions based actually in your specific scenario.

2. Pre-cutting-edge Medical Conditions: If you have have been given a pre-gift scientific scenario, which incorporates coronary heart illness, diabetes, arthritis, osteoporosis, or

some different continual contamination, you want to study how stretching sports activities may additionally have an impact in your health. When wearing out bodily sports activities, certain conditions may additionally moreover necessitate adaptations or unique care. A healthcare professional can advocate you on a manner to alter stretching wearing activities to fulfill your state of affairs and maintain you stable.

3. Harm Prevention: Consulting with a healthcare practitioner can lower the threat of harm extensively. They can study your musculoskeletal fitness and come across any areas of weakness, imbalances, or previous injuries that can necessitate greater care. You can study right techniques, adjustments, and progressions beneath professional supervision to avoid accidents and assure which you are completing stretches efficaciously.

four. Medication Considerations: If you take any drugs, you need to speak for your clinical physician approximately how they'll have an effect in your exercising addiction. Particular medicinal pills may additionally moreover additionally have horrible outcomes or interactions that could impair your functionality to carry out specific workout workouts or necessitate more precautions. Your healthcare provider can skip over your drug treatments with you and advocate you on any adjustments or issues to make at some point of your stretching habitual.

5. Improvement and Adjustments Monitoring: Regular appointments with a healthcare professional allow for persistent monitoring of your improvement. They may additionally display your flexibility, mobility, and ordinary fitness and make any modifications in your stretching exercise. They also can speak any issues or annoying situations you may be experiencing and offer pointers to help you efficiently triumph over them.

6. Holistic Approach to Health: Working with a healthcare expert offers for a greater

complete approach on your ordinary fitness and properly-being. They can endorse stretching sporting activities in addition to different factors of your way of life, collectively with vitamins, hydration, relaxation, and stress control. They can provide entire help to maximize your well-being by way of analyzing your normal health image.

7. Accountability and Motivation: Meeting with a healthcare corporation on a regular foundation gives a feel of responsibility and motivation. Knowing which you have an expert searching your development and helping your efforts may moreover assist you stay advocated to stick to your stretching software. It additionally lets in you to cope with any issues, challenges, or questions that may emerge, maintaining you on route closer to your goals.

Remember to the touch with a healthcare professional in case you are new to exercise, had been inactive for an prolonged period of time, or are having any health issues. They can provide you the self assurance and peace of thoughts to embark for your stretching adventure, know-how which you are prioritizing your health and protection.

Before starting a stretching exercise plan, talk over with a healthcare practitioner. Their know-how, tailor-made advice, and continuing help will let you keep away from accidents, deal with medical issues, tune development, and enhance your everyday nicely-being. This important segment guarantees that your stretching software is stable, powerful, and proper in your precise desires.

Setting Realistic Goals and Expectations

Setting low-cost goals and expectancies for oneself is crucial on the same time as beginning a stretching workout recurring. You can ensure a pleased and satisfying revel in in your journey to higher flexibility, mobility, and commonplace well-being by way of the use of doing so. Here are a few critical problems to maintain in thoughts even as creating goals and dealing with expectations:

1. Evaluate Your Current Fitness Level: Begin thru evaluating your modern-day fitness diploma and expertise your body's functionality. Think approximately your flexibility, range of motion, and regular bodily fitness. This self-evaluation will help you in setting up a baseline and identifying regions for increase.

2. Determining Your Motivation: Determine why you need to consist of stretching physical sports for your program. Is it to reduce joint stiffness, beautify posture, increase athletic basic overall performance, or absolutely promote extremely-modern-day fitness and properly-being? Understanding your motivation will help you in establishing huge and applicable desires.

three. Express and quantifiable Objectives: Establish specific and quantifiable dreams that may be tracked and assessed. Instead of a popular objective like "I need to be extra bendy," make it extra particular through using aiming to effects touch your feet or decorate your kind of movement in a particular joint. This permits you to diploma your development and function fun your accomplishments as you move.

4. Gradual Progression: Recognize that enhancing flexibility and mobility takes time and steady try. Avoid the need to hasten the method. Begin with mild stretching carrying activities and step by step increase the intensity, length, and complexity of the actions as your body becomes more acclimated to them. This slow method reduces the chance of damage and permits your body to regulate efficaciously.

Chapter 20: Essential Techniques And Principles

Importance of Proper Form and Alignment

One of the maximum important factors to don't forget at the equal time as performing stretching wearing sports is proper shape and alignment. It is critical to ensure which you do each stretch effectively and keep right posture in a few unspecified time inside the destiny of to maximize the advantages and reduce the hazard of harm. Here's why suitable form and alignment are important:

1. Targeting the Correct Muscles: Using proper form ensures which you are concentrated on the right muscle corporations for the stretch. Each stretch is supposed to stretch a selected muscle area, and using right shape permits isolate and have interaction those muscle tissue maximally. This permits a deeper and further powerful stretch, ensuing in accelerated flexibility and mobility.

2. Preventing Strains and Injuries: Poor shape and alignment can vicinity useless strain at the muscle companies, joints, and connective tissues, developing the danger of traces, sprains, and distinct accidents. Maintaining top alignment distributes the load in addition at some point of the body, lowering stress on any precise area. This encourages a extra steady stretching experience and reduces the possibility of overstretching or inflicting unneeded damage.

three. Improving Balance and Stability: Good shape and alignment in the course of stretching wearing sports help with stability and balance. By flawlessly aligning the frame's severa segments, you may construct a enterprise basis and boom proprioception, or the frame's revel in of spatial attention and region. This improves balance throughout stretches, decreasing the threat of falling or dropping stability.

4. Increasing Range of Motion: Proper shape and alignment permit you to boom your

shape of movement. Maintaining pinnacle-rated alignment lets in your joints to move through their complete style of movement, improving joint health and versatility. Moving inner a steady and cushty variety allows you to grade by grade increase your variety of motion over time with out producing undue pressure or soreness.

5. Improving Posture: Practicing appropriate form and alignment throughout stretching sports activities activities on a ordinary foundation helps enhance your widespread posture. Stretching lets in to prolong and loosen up tight muscle agencies, which can beautify alignment and accurate postural abnormalities. By efficiently aligning the body in a few unspecified time inside the future of stretches, you encourage healthier postural conduct throughout normal lifestyles.

6. Increasing Body Awareness: Focusing on properly form and alignment promotes frame focus. You construct a deeper reference to your body and its actions thru focusing on the

region of your body and the way it feels eventually of every stretch. This superior body recognition lets in you to make little tweaks and adjustments to guarantee splendid form, resulting in extra a success and more secure stretching periods.

7. Maximizing the Benefits: The closing motive of stretching carrying occasions is to gain their numerous blessings, which consist of accelerated flexibility, improved circulate, reduced muscle tension, and stepped forward big nicely-being. Proper form and alignment are critical for optimizing the ones advantages. Maintaining ok alignment allows muscles and connective tissues to stretch optimally, bearing in thoughts more will increase in flexibility and mobility.

www.ingramcontent.com/pod-product-compliance
Lightning Source LLC
Chambersburg PA
CBHW051728020426
42333CB00014B/1210